Peggy Munson
Editor

Stricken
Voices from the Hidden Epidemic of Chronic Fatigue Syndrome

Pre-publication
REVIEWS,
COMMENTARIES,
EVALUATIONS . . .

"**M**uch has been written about the physical impact of CFIDS, but far less about the destruction the illness wreaks upon the patient's life. *Stricken* provides a raw look at the personal stories of pain, isolation, and, ultimately, heroism of the millions worldwide who suffer from this complex illness."

Vicki Carpman Walker
Research and Public Policy
Project Manager,
The CFIDS Association of America

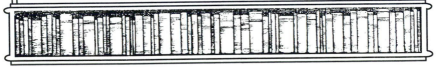

"**T**he aptly named *Stricken* is by turns a fact-filled, heart-wrenching, and sometimes hopeful book. It presents a mosaic of first-person narratives (from children and adolescents, as well as adults; from the most profound cases to those bordering on remission), plus poetry and essays about how the illness has been perceived over past decades. All those who have been felled by this indisputably 'hidden epidemic' will recognize their own experiences in these pages—a 'validating,' if sometimes downbeat, exercise, one that finally and definitively says they are not alone in their physical suffering. The book is also surprisingly up to date, including references to the most recent studies and theories about this so-far mysterious, but all-too-often devastating, disease.

The subtext of the book is also infuriating, when it touches on the way the medical community and the public at large have trivialized this genuinely disabling illness as 'yuppie flu,' 'psychoneurosis,' or 'mass hysteria.' Even many well-meaning clinicians, failing to recognize the most advanced cancer symptoms in patients who already have 'too many symptoms'—in short, by not really listening or by not ordering up appropriate new tests—have left some CFIDS patients in life-and-death situations.

The overall impact of *Stricken* is self-recognition for ill readers, both reassuring and unsettling. It can also serve as a powerful eye-opener for those—family, friends, doctors—who truly don't 'get it' yet. I recommend *Stricken* as a must-read (take out your yellow highlighter, mark it up, and then pass it along to those who still want to understand, regardless of how long you've been trying to explain what is basically an inexplicable disease). While I think I've read every related book on the market, this is the single best book I've read that honestly and fully describes the CFIDS experience."

Joan S. Livingston
Board of Directors,
Massachusetts CFIDS Association

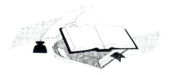

"**I**n *Stricken,* Munson educates the reader with her own informational narrative and through the personal accounts of persons with severe chronic fatigue syndrome who relate their struggles with this poorly understood yet devastating disorder, a serious illness with a silly trivializing name. CFS is an illness of numerous puzzling and often unpredictable symptoms. It affects the psyche, soma, and spirit, unraveling the fabric and quality of life, leaving no facet unaffected.

The voices of these sufferers with severe CFS are angry, pained, philosophical, needy, and insistent. Emanating from the CFS 'underground,' the authors display the otherwise invisible details and struggles of their own lives. Their desperation presents a vivid contrast to the public personae adopted so that one can 'pass' as well, to be socially acceptable in a world that frowns upon those who are severely, but invisibly, ill.

These courageous individuals relate stories that may seem exaggerated or even fabricated to the uninitiated, presenting a personal depth that is not conveyed through media or government accounts of CFS. It is indeed difficult for the healthy population to conceive that PWCs may appear perfectly healthy, while often lacking the energy, ability, and stamina to brush their teeth or bathe regularly, who can no longer read the morning newspaper, or follow the plot of a TV show. *Stricken* provides a vehicle for the voices of patients in isolation—their struggles, despair, fears—and simple joys."

Katrina Berne, PhD
Clinical Psychologist;
Author of *Running on Empty: The Complete Guide to Chronic Fatigue Syndrome (CFIDS)*

The Haworth Press, Inc.

Stricken
Voices from the Hidden Epidemic of Chronic Fatigue Syndrome

THE HAWORTH PRESS
New, Recent, and Forthcoming Titles
of Related Interest

Stricken
Voices from the Hidden Epidemic of Chronic Fatigue Syndrome

Peggy Munson
Editor

The Haworth Press®
New York • London • Oxford

The Haworth Press, Inc., 10 Alice Street, Binghamton, NY 13904-1580

Cover design by Monica Seifert.

Library of Congress Cataloging-in-Publication Data

Stricken : voices from the hidden epidemic of chronic fatigue syndrome / [edited by] Peggy Munson.
    p.   cm.
  Includes bibliographical references and index.
  ISBN 0-7890-0894-7 (hard : alk. paper)—ISBN 0-7890-0895-5 (soft : alk. paper)
  1. Chronic fatigue syndrome. I. Munson, Peggy.

RB150.F37 S77 2000
616′.0478—dc21
                                                            00-031930
                                                                  CIP

This book is for my family
and the loved ones of those in these pages.

And what I see sometimes is not the dark. But sometimes what I think I see is light. And I believe, no matter what I know, there is a light and I believe that I will see it some. And I believe that this will not endure forever, no, though for the time forseeable. But I believe that there will come a time when belt and boards will be undone, will loosen, and what holds me down, what keeps me here, will fall away . . .

Rebecca Brown
What Keeps Me Here

CONTENTS

ABOUT THE EDITOR

Peggy Munson is an award-winning fiction writer, poet, and essayist whose recent work has appeared in such places as *Literature and Medicine,* the *Spoon River Poetry Review, 13th Moon, The San Francisco Bay Guardian,* and in anthologies published by Faber and Faber, Cleis Press, and Creative Arts Book Company.

Ms. Munson has been awarded fellowships at the MacDowell Colony, the Ragdale Foundation, and Cottages at Hedgebrook, and holds a degree in Creative Writing from Oberlin College. Though she suffered from pre-onset symptoms, she became severely ill with CFIDS in 1992, following a sudden infection. For several years, she was an active organizer and support leader in the online CFIDS community. She is a Midwest native who now makes her home in New England.

CONTRIBUTORS

Kathleen Bogan is an attorney and visual artist as well as a poet. Her work, which has won many prizes, appears in journals including *Confrontation, Seattle Review, Atlanta Review, Writers' Forum, Earth's Daughters* and many others, and the anthologies *The Muse Strikes Back, Prairie Hearts: Women Writers Writing About the Midwest,* and *Sirius Verse.* She contracted CFIDS following a trip to East Africa in 1987, and her health forced her to retire from work as a national criminal justice policy consultant and Oregon state agency head in 1992. Her home is in Portland, Oregon.

Andrew Corriveau is a freelance writer living on the East Coast. He encourages all able-bodied people to confront their own fears and to get involved in CFIDS activism.

Susan Dion, PhD, has received four Puffin Foundation grants to fund WRITE NOW, a free resource on coping with illness. She slowly writes about women's issues, education, disability/illness concerns, coping, and other topics. In 1999, her poems, essays, and reviews were included in several publications. She's written many articles for CFIDS journals and newsletters. The essay "Sick Sex" (which inspired "Sick Sex Revisited") was originally published by the Connecticut CFIDS Association in the Spring 1994 *Network.*

Kat Duff is an astrological counselor and author. Her book, *The Alchemy of Illness,* is available from Bell Tower Books. "The Dark Heart of Healing," a two-cassette-tape set based on the book, is available from Sounds True. Her essays have appeared in *Parabola* magazine.

Eva Marie Everson is married, has three children, and lives in Orlando, Florida, where she currently writes for several ministries and publications. Eva is the co-author of *Pinches of Salt, Prisms of Light.* She is a contributing author to works by Lynn Morrissey and Kathy Collard Miller, an active speaker and teacher, and is working on her second novel and a gift book.

Kate Foran is currently a student at Manchester Community College. She was a recipient of MCC's Outstanding Young Poet award in 1998. Last spring, she was chosen to tour on the Connecticut Poetry Circuit as a Connecticut Student Poet. Her work has been published in literary journals such as *Skywriters, Shapes,* and *Common Ground Review.* She's grateful for her CFIDS experience, which has taught her to pay attention to her body, as well as to the world around her.

Before CFIDS, **Nadine Goranson** worked full-time, including work as a writing teacher, helping senior citizens to write their life stories. Diagnosed with CFIDS in 1994, she now spends her time caring for her family, reading, writing, and resting with her dog, Sammy, near the Rocky Mountains of Colorado.

Susan Griffin is a writer, poet, essayist, lecturer, teacher, filmmaker, and Emmy-winning playwright. She was named by *Utne Reader* as one of "100 Visionaries Who Could Change Your Life." Author of the Pulitzer Prize-nominated *A Chorus of Stones,* as well as the best-selling *Woman and Nature, Pornography and Silence,* and *The Eros of Everyday Life,* Griffin's latest books are *What Her Body Thought,* from which this excerpt is taken, and *Bending Home: New and Selected Poems.*

Phyllis Griffiths lives in Victoria, British Columbia, Canada. She holds a BA from the University of Lethbridge in the field of anthropology, which she put to use doing Heritage Conservation and museum management before becoming severely disabled by CFIDS in late 1990. Over the years her family has helped many street kids to get off the streets and has developed a large extended family. Currently Phyllis is active via the Internet, where she has placed the manuscript "Valley of Shadows" on her personal Web site. She also has been active as an e-mail support group leader and CFIDS activist as her health allows.

Gloria Kartiganer is an educator working on school reform and is a theater artist; eager to find a group to join in education and action for CFIDS; please reach her at <spicecarrier@yahoo.com>.

Dorian Key is a boy-identified dyke who lives in the Bay Area. Her work appears in *Best Lesbian Erotica 1998, Wicked Women, On Our Backs,* and *Strategic Sex.*

Mayra Lazara was born in Marianao, Cuba, grew up in Hialeah, Florida, and lived in Boston throughout her twenties. She's worked as a hairstylist and landscape designer. This is her first published piece. Due to the severity of her illness, she spends her time writing and has recently finished a humorous fiction manuscript.

Caitlin MacEwan is the pseudonym of a writer with CFIDS. Under her real name, she has published articles, essays, poetry, drawings, and satire internationally, primarily in Neopagan and feminist journals. She is a priestess in an Ecofeminist Celtic Reconstructionist Pagan tradition and a founding member of a number of spiritual circles and organizations. She is a proud veteran of ACT UP and other radical direct-action groups, and believes that spirituality and political activism go hand in hand. In younger, healthier days, she also performed and recorded magical music with a womyn's band. She has struggled with gradual-onset CFIDS, MCS, and varying levels of disability for most of her life.

Stacey Montgomery lives by her wits in the Jamaica Plain end of Boston. She spends her time writing, designing interactivity, and being Femme Mommie to the Lesbian Avengers of Boston. She's still hoping that she will end up a supermodel or a superhero. This is her first published poem.

Mary Munson is a former educator, newspaper reporter, and health food store owner. She has corenovated numerous historic buildings. She lives in the Midwest.

Joan Nestle is a pioneering activist in the feminist and lesbian communities. Born in New York City in 1940, a working-class Jew raised by her mother, Nestle was at the forefront of pivotal political actions, helping to establish the Gay Academic Union and later, the Lesbian Herstory Archives, which now fill a three-story building in Park Slope, Brooklyn. She is the author of *A Fragile Union* and *A Restricted Country,* and editor of *The Persistent Desire: A Femme-Butch Reader* and *Sister and Brother: Lesbians and Gay Men Write About Their Lives Together.* She is also the co-editor of *The Vintage Book of International Lesbian Fiction* and the *Women on Women Anthologies of American Lesbian Short Fiction.* She has won many awards, including the Bill Whitehead Award for Lifetime Achievement in Lesbian and Gay Literature, American Library Association Gay/Lesbian Book Award, and the Lambda Literary Award.

Gary Null, PhD, is an award-winning journalist and author of dozens of books including *Gary Null's Ultimate Anti-Aging Program, Healing Your Body Naturally, Change Your Life Now,* and *The Healthy Body Book.* A prominent health advocate and broadcast journalist, he has also been a guest on talk shows such as *Oprah, Donahue,* and *Letterman.* He is the host of the nationally syndicated *The Gary Null Health and Nutrition Program,* and has educated thousands of people on environmental hazards, the interplay of chemicals in our lives, sensible nutrition, and healing.

James Rotholz, PhD, lives in Maryland with his wife and children. They have worked with relief and development programs in Ethiopia, Somalia, and Nepal. Before contracting CFIDS, Dr. Rotholz was Assistant Professor of anthropology at Washington State University. His chapter is revised from an unpublished book on Christianity, culture, and CFIDS.

Ellen Samuels' poetry and essays have recently appeared in *Kalliope, The American Voice, Journal of the American Medical Association,* and the anthology *Lesbians, Levis, & Lipstick.* She also co-edited *Out of the Ordinary: Reflections on Growing Up with Lesbian, Gay, Bisexual & Transgender Parents* (St. Martin's Press). Ellen has earned degrees from Oberlin College and Cornell University, and now lives in Berkeley, CA. She has been ill since 1995.

Floyd Skloot is the author of three novels and two collections of poetry. His book of essays about the illness experience, *The Night Side* (Story Line Press, 1996) was named one of the best books of the season by *New Age Journal.* Skloot's writing about illness has been reprinted in *The Best American Essays of 1993* and *The Art of the Essay 1999* as well as in such journals as *The American Scholar, Commonweal, Boulevard, Antioch Review, Southwest Review, Missouri Review,* and many others. He lives in Amity, Oregon, with his wife Beverly Hallberg.

June Stein wants to use her biography space to plead to all healthy folks reading this essay: "We need you in our activism! We can't do it without you!"

In the earliest years of CFIDS-related illness, **Chris Szabo** used writing for recreation. Following encouragement from editors and publishers, Chris wrote for *Armoured Fighting Vehicle News* and other military-related magazines, including a main feature in *Air Enthusiast,* and a column in the specialist Balkan magazine, *Delusions of Grandeur.*

Dorothy Wall is co-author of *Finding Your Writer's Voice: A Guide to Creative Fiction* (St. Martin's Press, 1994). She has taught poetry and fiction writing at San Francisco State University, Napa Valley College, and UC Berkeley, Extension, and is a writing consultant in Berkeley. Her health is steadily improving.

Willy Wilkinson is a writer and public health consultant. She has written for a number of publications, including *Curve, Sojourner,* and the *San Francisco Bay Times.* Her piece "Remember the Place Where Your Soul Lives: Chronic Fatigue Immune Dysfunction Syndrome" in *The Lesbian Health Book* (Seal Press, 1997) highlighted the issue of CFIDS in the lesbian community. Other anthologies in which her work has appeared include *The Gender Politics of HIV/AIDS in Women: Perspectives on the Pandemic in the United States* (New York University Press, 1997) and *The Very Inside: An Anthology of Writing by Asian and Pacific Islander Lesbian and Bisexual Women* (Sister Vision Press, 1994). She lives with her beautiful, irreverent wife Georgia in Oakland, California.

Foreword

A choice that confronts every one of us encountering the voices of those with chronic fatigue immune dysfunction syndrome (CFIDS) is this: Shall we permit ourselves to know and accept these voices as they are, or shall we remain estranged observers, forever labeling, judging, and placing blame? This choice has always been available, but the majority of us have failed to listen to and wholly understand the authenticity of these voices and the relentless pain rendered by CFIDS. Camouflaged and silenced, these voices cannot be whole without the courage to be known in simple honesty.

Through her compilation of vivid and poignant writings, Peggy Munson frees some of these voices to provide an intimate view into life in the world of those with CFIDS; life likened to an ugly death by some, as well as to a rebirth of the human spirit through creativity, self-recollection, and the reconstruction of a psychological sense of community by others. Faced with devastating symptoms and multiple losses, the voices of those with CFIDS reveal beauties and strengths associated with the intangibles of human existence—love, community, and self-discovery. With new meaning, direction, and purpose, these voices have found a way to be heard. With strength and matchless bravery, they have found a way to reshape our conceptualizations of individuals with CFIDS, so that the world may be more equipped to handle the complexity of this chronic illness.

One of the most devastating issues facing individuals with CFIDS is public, familial, and professional skepticism about the reality of "invisible" symptoms and impairments. As captured in the essay by Dorothy Wall, "Encounters with the Invisible," denial of the reality of CFIDS by the external world can sometimes give way to self-denial and self-estrangement, both having devastating consequences to the wholeness and stability that are so crucial to inner healing. Negative attitudes toward individuals with CFIDS may, in part, be a function of past government and media portrayals of these illnesses as either nonexistent or as a function of a neurotic, overworked, stressed lifestyle, as was depicted in the popular media label for CFIDS, "yuppie flu." Such media portrayals hold individuals responsible for their illness and therefore ignore illness givens associated with the unfairness, fragility, and unpredictability of human existence. This phenomenon of victim blaming is reflected in the fundamental attribution error known as "belief in a just world," the belief that life "justly" rewards or punishes people for their actions through good or bad fortune.

In addition, there has been considerable controversy over the term, chronic fatigue syndrome, used to describe the illness. Patient advocacy groups contend that this name tends to minimize the seriousness and complexity of the illness, and recent research supports this argument.[1,2] Findings from two studies have indicated that the name chronic fatigue syndrome may be regarded less seriously than the name myalgic encephalopathy (often proposed as an alternate term for CFIDS) with respect to some important aspects of the illness, including attributions regarding illness cause. The term myalgic encephalopathy was significantly more likely than chronic fatigue syndrome to prompt attributions to a medical cause, rather than a psychiatric cause.

In our efforts to better understand people's attitudes toward individuals with CFIDS, our research team at DePaul University developed the Chronic Fatigue Syndrome Attitudes Test (CAT).[3] It is a valid and reliable measure designed to assess knowledge and attributions regarding CFIDS among individuals who do not have CFIDS. This nineteen-item scale was created using several constructs outlined in the literature regarding negative attitudes toward people with CFIDS, other disabilities, and AIDS. The results of a study with the CAT revealed a relationship between beliefs about the degree to which people with CFIDS are responsible for their illness, beliefs about the relevance of CFIDS as a valid illness, and beliefs about the personality traits of people with CFIDS. If someone believes that people with CFIDS are responsible for their illness, it is likely that they will also believe that people with CFIDS have negative personality characteristics, such as being compulsive or overly driven.

A second theme uniting the voices in this anthology involves an overwhelming lack of community responsiveness to the illness. People with CFIDS are at once both severely functionally impaired and very underserved, yet they are not currently recognized as either by most medical and community-based service programs. As a result of this tension between impaired persons with CFIDS and a lack of socioenvironmental responsiveness, persons with CFIDS are among the most disabled of those with chronic illness. Historically, individuals with CFIDS have been underserved for five reasons: (1) the disability has drained them of all or almost all economic and social resources and has left a majority unemployed or further disabled by their employment situation; (2) those with fewest resources are under severe economic hardship, isolated, and unable to provide for their own housing; (3) those who are unable to work have had tremendous difficulty obtaining Social Security and disability benefits to help subsidize their income, in spite of the fact that the Social Security Administration recognizes CFIDS as a disability; (4) many treatments attempted by individuals with CFIDS do not work and are, at best, palliative for isolated symptoms; (5) as a result of being misdiagnosed with primary psychiatric disorders by physicians, invalidated by co-workers, friends, and family, and frequently turned down by community agencies for benefits received by individuals with other disabilities, the illness experience of those with CFIDS is often compounded by this societal iatrogenesis.

Inspiration, psychological resiliency, a sense of community through sharing, and hope constitute a third central theme of this anthology. In the words of Floyd Skloot, "By telling [my story of CFIDS] more widely, I am not only helping myself remember, I am bearing witness, and trying to reclaim my humanity, bringing it out of the shadows of lost memories and into the light of experience." Similarly, Peggy Munson's essay, "On Life, Death, and the Nature of Limbo," shares how the development of a sense of community can occur through writing. Munson's essay describes the value in understanding and appreciating life *as the limbo,* and in respecting beauty and stability found within the present moment. It communicates hope in confronting the erratic and startling swings of CFIDS symptomatology through embracing one's spirit and body *as they are,* and through accepting and appreciating help, understanding, and support from caring others.

In an attempt to map out a schema for psychological and social adaptation to the startling and unusual symptoms and illness severity flux characteristic of CFIDS, we worked with Patricia Fennell to develop the Fennell Phases Inventory. The Fennell Phases Inventory, a twenty-item questionnaire, is a promising way of differentiating among four different phases that are experienced by individuals with CFIDS.[4] The four phases measured by this inventory include: crisis, stabilization, resolution, and integration.[5] In phase 1, the crisis phase, individuals move from the initial onset of CFIDS to an eventual crisis state, wherein they respond with uncertainty and emotional distress to the trauma of a new illness. In phase 2, the stabilization phase, individuals continue to experience physical and behavioral chaos, followed by an eventual stabilization characterized by some recognition and predictability of their symptoms. In phase 3, the resolution phase, individuals work to accept the chronicity and ambiguity of the illness and create meaning out of the illness experience. Phase 3 is characterized by plateau, relapse, or progression, all constituting the normal cycling of chronic illness. In the final stage, the integration phase, individuals advance to a state of integration, where they are able to integrate pre- and post-illness self-concepts and sometimes psychologically transcend the CFIDS illness. They realize they may either continue to cycle, or their health may improve significantly. Patients often construct a new identity; a combination of themselves before and after the illness experience. In sum, the Fennell phases model and Fennell Phases Inventory[6] emphasize that individuals with CFIDS can achieve a sense of psychological, social, and emotional mastery over the illness, regardless of the body's physical condition and functioning.

From Munson's collection of essays, the importance of maintaining a psychological sense of community, a feeling of connectedness, reciprocity, and identification with the collective other, is strikingly apparent. A bitter reality facing many with CFIDS is the violation of the sense of community that was once present in their lives before illness onset. How can replenishment of a sense of community be actualized? To date, effective, affordable, comprehensive assessment and treatment programs do not exist to address both the medical and social service needs of individuals with CFIDS. Thus, there is a clear need for programs in which people can be individually assessed, treatment can be specifically tailored to meet the unique needs of individuals with CFIDS, and individuals with CFIDS can come together to benefit from mutual emotional and informational support. Ultimately, such programs would enhance the welfare of individuals both directly, through their participation in services, and indirectly, through dissemination, program replication, and public education, all contributing to a potential for increased allocation of resources to individuals with CFIDS.

A vision for such a program is that it would provide a thorough and individualized assessment, which would lead to access to medical and social services provided by practitioners specializing in CFIDS. A comprehensive treatment plan would be developed for each client based on that individual's need. This might include focusing on increasing physical, occupational, social, and/or psychological functioning. The program would also provide resources to educate clients and their families about CFIDS. Based on individual needs, the program would link clients with needed resources such as financial assistance, housing, and personal assistance for activities of daily living. Emphasis would be placed on providing clients with a support network of similar others, and with linkage to educated and effective service providers. Clients would become self-empowered by actively participating in activities of the comprehensive center. Services available through the program would be developed through the collaboration of on-site and local health and social service professionals, in conjunction with experts in the area of CFIDS, and with guidance from local and national CFIDS self-help organizations.

The program would also provide advocacy services, including educating the public, and particularly medical and vocational service providers, about the nature and treatment of these conditions, and about the services offered by the program. The program would work toward social policy change at a higher level, increasing, by its requests on behalf of patients, the provision of effective services and resources. These efforts would increase acceptance and acknowledgment of these conditions, and the public, both general and medical, would become more responsive to the needs of individuals with CFIDS.

With hope for continued exemplars of community building among individuals with CFIDS, Munson's valuable work encompasses its own community of voices portraying a multifaceted narrative of the CFIDS experience. We consider ourselves most fortunate to have been selected to bear witness to the courage, personal struggles, and inner accomplishments depicted within this volume. We have witnessed remarkable strength, coping, and resilience among those who have shared their experiences in these pages. As a point of departure for future research, this anthology leads us to cast strong doubt on the capacity of most research to adequately represent those most debilitated by this illness. Akin to the experiences shared in this volume, many individuals with CFIDS are so disabled that it is impossible for them to even move from a bed for prolonged periods of time. Thus, it is highly likely that research based on laboratory or medical clinic studies of individuals with CFIDS excludes individuals most in need of representation and most in need of services. To the extent possible, we strongly recommend that future research employ community-based strategies when attempting to fully understand and provide recommendations for individuals with CFIDS. Such strategies serve to more accurately represent the true voices of those with CFIDS.

Leonard A. Jason, PhD
DePaul University

Renée R. Taylor, PhD
DePaul University

NOTES

1. Jason, L.A., Taylor, R.R., Plioplys, S., Stepanek, Z., and Shlaes, J. (in press). Evaluating attributions for an illness based upon the name: Chronic fatigue syndrome, myalgic encephalopathy, and Florence Nightingale disease. *American Journal of Community Psychology*.

2. Jason, L.A., Taylor, R.R., Stepanek, Z., and Plioplys, S. (1999). *Attitudes regarding chronic fatigue syndrome: The importance of a name*. Manuscript submitted for publication.

3. Shlaes, J.L., Jason, L.A., and Ferrari, J.R. (1999). The development of the chronic fatigue syndrome attitudes test. *Evaluation and the Health Professions*, 22(4), 442–465.

4. Jason, L.A., Fennell, P.A., Klein, S., Fricano, G., Halpert, J.A., and Taylor, R.R. (1999). An investigation of the different phases of the CFS illness. *Journal of Chronic Fatigue Syndrome*, 5(3/4), 35-54.

5. Fennell, P.A. (1993). A systematic, four-stage progressive model for mapping the CFIDS experience. *The CFIDS Chronicle*, Summer, 40-46.

6. Jason, L.A., Fennell, P.A., Klein, S., Fricano, G., Halpert, J.A., and Taylor, R.R. (1999). An investigation of the different phases of the CFS illness. *Journal of Chronic Fatigue Syndrome*, 5(3/4), 35-54.

Preface

Imagine if your entire well-being depended on the telling of a story. Chances are, at some point in time, it will.

Because you are mortal, because your mortal body fails, you will stand at the gates of medicine and society, wearing a baggy robe much like the loose garb of a chain gang as you plead for consideration. Someone will scribe notes about your most personal details—the fact that you are black, nervous, gay, impotent, constipated, scared—which may be used to prove or disprove your diagnosis. Someone may see your story as a parable, a lie, an impossibility. If you become sick to the point of being disabled, you will need a lawyer, in addition to expert witnesses, to prove you have told the whole truth. Many times, in many places, you will feel like a criminal for what you wish for, for what you are.

Some skeptics may look for emotional pathology among these pages. They may only see suicidal thoughts, spiritual critique, political ravings. But in this set of stories, there will be moments of transgression. These are human stories, intricate struggles, and not just clinical tales with neat empirical margins. They are stories of the lives of a diverse population, people united by the unnamed pathogen that has pushed them underground. They are tales of grief and hope. And within these pages, within the lives of the stricken, lies the complex truth.

Acknowledgments

This book would not have been finished without the gracious support of many people, and to those I would like to offer my gratitude. To the friends who gave me practical and emotional support, and especially to Rachel Samet for her enormous heart, and Abe Doherty for meals, laughter, and tears. To Mom, for helping me edit, being a careful reader, and being an amazing role model. To Dad, for CFIDS activism over the airwaves and so much more. To Molly, my big sister, for driving miles to provide assistance, and always being my ally and good friend. To Mayra Lazara, for honesty and eloquence, and for prodding me with exclamation points until I started this book. To other friends who have shared the illness journey with me as I worked on this book: Jody Schutz, Michael Druzinsky, Nina McIntosh, Toni Amato, Amy Aisenberg, Sharon Wachsler, and Janet Hyland. To the great folks I met at QCFS: Buffalo, Moe, Florrie, Kathryn, and all the others. To Bob Barsy for help with the foreword. For last-minute research help, thanks to Chuck Diesel and Gitana Garafolo. To the contributors in this book, many of whom have become friends, for being an editor's dream cast.

Also, kudos to the renegade doctors and healers who stood by their patients in the face of opposition and cultural prejudice, and to the CFIDS writers and activists who have raised awareness. To the many others with this illness who have touched my life, both as friends and acquaintances. To my wonderful readers: Rob McDale, Mari McKeeth, and Sandy Bush. To the Ragdale Foundation and Cottages at Hedgebrook for residences that nurtured me as a writer. To my doctors and healers, with special thanks to Dr. Mark Brody and Jay Minkin. To Oberlin College for making me an activist. Last, to my gentle canine companion, Rowley, who helped me appreciate the simple things.

Introduction

Peggy Munson

Several years ago, a group of neuropsychologists published a study correlating the fragmented writing style of a subset of nuns with their higher incidence of Alzheimer's disease later in life. Looking at early school writing samples from over 700 retired Midwestern nuns, they found that young novices who wrote biographical essays in very simple sentences later perished with symptoms of Alzheimer's, whereas those with more complex prose styles did not.[1]

When I began editing *Stricken,* I became painfully aware of the ways chronic fatigue immune dysfunction syndrome (CFIDS) also undermines the linguistic process and defeats the efforts of people with CFIDS (PWCs) to convey their own hermetic world. CFIDS is a multisystemic disease that, among other things, leads to severe cognitive problems such as memory loss and word-finding difficulties. One remarkable study, utilizing specific brain scan techniques, found the effects of CFIDS on the brain to be strikingly similar to those of AIDS dementia.[2] Earlier research discovered punctate lesions in CFIDS brains resembling those of multiple sclerosis patients.[3] Dr. Paul Cheney found that in dual chromatography analyses, many CFIDS patients actually had more derangement of the brain, on a biochemical level, than Parkinson's or Alzheimer's patients.[4] Dr. Sheila Bastien, who studied a group of educated patients, was stunned to realize that patients who initially appeared very lucid had suffered tremendous drops in IQ points, so severe in some cases that "a few performance IQs were startlingly close to the legal definition of idiocy."[5] Thus, as I culled submissions, writers with higher education degrees sent me notes apologizing for their choppy sentences. Published poets told me the subject matter of their own illness was too painful, too difficult to convey. Reliable literary friends promised to write me pieces and then sent frantic e-mails saying they were bed bound, having a severe relapse, or too brain-fogged to begin. One writer—in a classic CFIDS haze—actually mailed me her medication schedule. Often, I wished I were editing a book on, say, workaholism or hypermania. I felt like the editorial Cruella De Vil.

As a seven-year CFIDS sufferer and published writer, I knew how much the very act of writing, the laborious mental output, even the exertion of putting a submission in an envelope or licking a stamp, depleted so many of those who sent work. As I edited this book, I was almost completely homebound, sick beyond my wildest imagination, and struggling every minute myself. I came to understand the dearth of first-person CFIDS narratives and the contrasting abundance of misinformed articles speaking for the ill population. One writer who had largely recovered gently refused my request to anthologize a previously published piece of his, since he didn't want his painful and inchoate experience immortalized. His anxiety was especially touching in this epidemic of public paranoia, in which words have been given extreme diagnostic power and many have implied infection can happen with the mere uttering of a name. In the absence of first-person narratives, chronic fatigue syndrome quickly became perceived as a disease of cultural incantation, the patients seen as suggestible individuals under temporary hypnosis, a kind of cult.

CFIDS patients have been pushed underground not only by the circumscription of illness, but by jeering criticism about the legitimacy of their diagnosis. If a simple writing style can predict incidence of neurological decay, as the Alzheimer's study suggests, what other roles might language play in illness and its public perception? As Western doctors banter around terms such as "cell memory," attributing a personality to the organs, and Eastern medicine influences our notions of the emotional qualities of the viscera, stories indeed play a growing role in our understanding of body processes. Can hateful words rallied against a disabled population, like the hypothesized infrasonic damage from an earthquake miles away, cause physical injury? Can the story of an illness be properly told when its sufferers can only speak or write in halting sentences, or when they are too sick to communicate outside of their own homes? Can writing about physical ailments, as one study in the *Journal of the American Medical Association* suggests, actually help lessen the severity of a patient's symptoms?[6] *Stricken* is not only a collection of literary writings about the CFIDS epidemic, but a critique of the mythology and language surrounding an illness population and a collection of its untold stories.

Stricken comes at the crux of some riveting literary and political trends. The "man versus nature" narrative has become increasingly popular at the turn of the millennium, with best-sellers such as *Into Thin Air* and *The Hot Zone.* Meanwhile, with the rise of the trash psychology of TV talk shows, laypeople have endowed themselves with diagnostic power and spoken out loudly against the CFIDS population. Rush Limbaugh, *The Wall Street Journal,* and even the government's appointed expert on CFIDS, Stephen Straus, have all taken insensitive potshots against those stricken with this disease. Nobody has partaken in such a zealous barrage of metaphoric lampoons since the nineteenth century days of multiple sclerosis, which was called in its early years "hysterical paralysis."

Ultimately, despite the strict diagnostic parameters that left little doubt about the devastation of CFIDS, the portrayal of the illness degenerated into name calling. The "yuppie flu" tagline for CFIDS, which emerged in the 1980s, paved the way for the 1990s decrier Elaine Showalter, a Princeton feminist literary critic with a self-proclaimed love of bargain shopping. Safely out of the clutches of Susan Sontag's *Illness As Metaphor,* which forced literary scholars to examine the way cultural metaphors distort true suffering, Showalter found her sale of the century in CFIDS, a disease swarming with inaccurate metaphors and simplistic cultural interpretations. Her 1997 book *Hystories: Hysterical Epidemics and Modern Media* called CFIDS one of the major hysterical epidemics of the late twentieth century. After an extensive book tour that included talk show spots and supposed death threats that seemed to boost her public credibility, Showalter was named president of the prestigious Modern Languages Association. This seemed a startling accolade for a professor who based her own scholarship almost entirely on popular magazine articles, yet critiqued the way people mimic pop culture by embodying accounts of illness.

A prevalence study released by the Centers for Disease Control (CDC) in 1998 announced that the incidence of CFIDS is now higher than that of lung cancer, breast cancer, or HIV infection in women,[7] but CFIDS had already been stricken from the government's agenda. Government CFIDS official William Reeves took a surprising turn that year, declaring under the immunity of the "whistle-blowers act" that most government CFIDS funds had been diverted into other accounts. In fact, an internal audit found that the CDC spent a large percentage of its already paltry CFIDS funding, from 1995 to 1998, on other diseases, then blatantly lied to Congress about these misappropriations.[8] Only a total of $23 million was allocated for CFIDS for those years to begin with, an astoundingly meager sum for an illness of this magnitude. Only $9.8 million of these funds were spent on CFIDS in a period during which Kenneth Starr spent $40 million of taxpayers' money to prove that *one* American president had sex with an intern.[9,10] The myopia of this fiscal distribution, in the face of an epidemic that could cripple the economy and public health, is astounding. William Reeves stated on CNN that this funding fiasco "probably set us back three to five years" in terms of government research and programs.[11] Although worldwide researchers were on the brink of breakthrough discoveries and potential diagnostic tests, and advocates were fighting hard for a more legitimate name for the illness, the government had even cancelled its funding for the first federally sponsored research into pediatric CFIDS.

At the turn of the millennium, the public still lacks a real grasp on what CFIDS patients are dealing with. Because of illusions that CFIDS is simply a disease of tired people, and not one that has left Olympic athletes such as Michelle Akers, Inga Thompson, and Amy Petersen immobilized, the public has been largely deprived of accurate information. As notoriously energetic jazz pianist Keith Jarrett, also stricken with the illness, put it, "It's stupid to call it Chronic Fatigue Syndrome. It should be called the forever dead syndrome."[12] One thing is certainly deceptive: CFIDS patients rarely look as sick as they are. Dr. Mark Loveless, an infectious disease specialist, proclaimed that a CFIDS patient "feels every day significantly the same as an AIDS patient feels two months before death."[13] People react to such severity with disbelief. *How,* they query, *could it be so bad if we haven't heard about it?* I would argue that the debilitating nature of the symptoms creates the pervasive silence, paving the way for a mythology that has haunted the epidemic since its inception.

The devastation of illness is hard to quantify, but some clinicians have tried. Dr. Dan Peterson, one of the doctors who delineated a tragic CFIDS cluster outbreak in Incline Village, Nevada (often considered the epicenter of the disease), employed a protocol called the Medical Outcome Study to systematically evaluate the level of suffering in a group of CFIDS patients. He and his colleagues measured people with CFIDS against a control group and against patients with various ailments. When he presented his findings, Peterson revealed the astonishing fact that no other set of patients had ever measured so poorly. CFIDS patients experienced greater "functional severity" than the studied patients with heart disease, virtually all types of cancer, and all other chronic illnesses.[14] An unrelated study compared the quality of life of people with various illnesses, including patients undergoing chemotherapy or hemodialysis, as well as those with HIV, liver transplants, coronary artery disease, and other ailments, and again found that CFIDS patients scored the lowest.[15] "In other words," said Dr. Leonard Jason in a radio interview, "this disease, this syndrome, is actually more debilitating than just about any other kind of medical problem in the world."[16] Nevertheless, most accounts of the illness have simply shortened its name to the flip and damaging misnomer "chronic fatigue" as if CFIDS is a mild inconvenience. Chronic fatigue is actually an entirely different condition from CFIDS, a symptom of many illnesses or a result of overexertion, affecting up to a quarter of the population.[17] CFIDS, like all illnesses, strikes on a continuum of severity, in some cases with fluctuating periods of relapse and remission. And of course, a percentage of patients do recover partially or fully, though "recovery" from CFIDS has been poorly defined, and in fact often appears to be more of a remission. When asked on CNN how many of his CFIDS patients had *fully* recovered in fifteen years, Dr. Peterson unequivocally and chillingly stated, "None."[18] Most CFIDS patients, tragically, are far too sick to tell their own stories or to fight the pervasive ignorance about their condition. The politics of CFIDS still possess a kind of insularity.

Telling the stories of this epidemic still seems to be a radical act. As I plowed through recent articles about CFIDS, I discovered a biased media that favors a nonmedical, almost metaphorical approach to the illness. In a July 9, 1999, search of *The New York*

Times Web site, which posts several years of articles, I found twenty-two that mentioned chronic fatigue syndrome. Of these, the majority included one-line citations of the illness in conjunction with other issues, such as underground drug sales or Lyme disease. Thirteen of the twenty-two spoke of CFIDS in reference to world-class soccer player and atypical CFIDS patient Michelle Akers (perhaps giving the misleading impression that the majority of CFIDS patients can win the World Cup, and prompting syndicated columnist Ellen Goodman to exclaim, "If that's chronic fatigue syndrome, how do I get it?"[19]). Keith Jarrett, much sicker than Akers, only got one article, perhaps because—as his agent said to me—Jarrett is generally too sick to do interviews. Three articles debated the legitimacy of the diagnosis or entertained hysteria theories. In fact, though *The New York Times* Web site mentioned CFIDS more than any other publication site I searched, actual coverage of it as a *medical illness* was appallingly neglectful. Not a *single* article of the twenty-two dealt with current CFIDS research, social issues related to the illness (such as the CDC scandal), the shocking new prevalence statistics, or anything remotely hopeful for CFIDS patients. In contrast, there were ample articles on other diseases—280 on a search of HIV, 98 for multiple sclerosis, 238 for lung cancer, and 400 for breast cancer. Many of these used medical lingo such as "Women and AIDS: The Better Half Got the Worse End," "Injection of Cells Aids Mice," and "Drug Slashes Breast Cancer Risk, Study Shows." But then, the only article in the twenty-two that was almost wholly about CFIDS was in the Arts section, a story about a speculative Internet musical exploring links between AIDS and CFIDS.[20]

This startling neglect fuels the vicious paradox of CFIDS. Although publications such as the *CFIDS Chronicle* and the *Journal of Chronic Fatigue Syndrome* detail hundreds of recognizable abnormalities in CFIDS patients, discovered through rigorous clinical research, CFIDS patients—shunned by doctors and the media and often their friends—are forced to go underground, adding to their own invisibility. The *Hartford Courant* noted that the CDC also cancelled educational efforts aimed at pediatricians and teachers, as well as research projects targeted at helping minorities and health workers with CFIDS.[21] With a little diligence, however, one can easily discover that CFIDS—like AIDS—is infiltrating the world in devastating ways. Long stereotyped as a disease of rich, white American women, one San Francisco CDC prevalence study found the highest prevalence of the illness in African-American and Native American populations.[22] A study in Chicago found that Latinos are at the highest risk for the illness, and that those in lower income brackets suffer from CFIDS disproportionately. In fact, contradicting the "yuppie flu" image, the researchers actually discovered that skilled craftspeople, clerical and sales workers, and machine operators are much more likely to get CFIDS, while higher-paid professionals have the lowest rates of the illness.[23] Dr. David Bell speculates in *The Doctor's Guide to Chronic Fatigue Syndrome* that people with CFIDS, deprived of health care and unable to keep their jobs, "may be a major contributor to the homeless problem in this country."[24] On the World Wide Web, I was able to find CFIDS Web sites in Great Britain, Canada, the Netherlands, Japan, Australia, Sweden, South Africa, Denmark, Argentina, and Israel—in other words, on every continent but Antarctica. Many offered impressive synopses of international research, showing that prominent researchers all over the globe—generally without the support of drug companies, governments, or publicity—are dedicating themselves to decrypting the mystery of this devastating disease. For researchers such as Dr. Nancy Klimas, studying CFIDS is an act of intrigue and self-sacrifice, or as she says in the book *Osler's Web,* "very interesting, fascinating, and completely unfunded work."[25]

Though many people with CFIDS have extreme difficulty obtaining disability benefits, claims related to the illness have skyrocketed. In 1985, Chicago philanthropist Ted Van Zelst commissioned an extensive study about CFIDS, which was completed in 1986. Forty percent of the CFIDS patients he studied were completely disabled by the disease. Nearly all of these said they had been denied Social Security benefits.[26] In 1995, things were not much better—only 14.5 percent of CFIDS claims got initial approval for Social Security Disability Income, compared with a 30.9 percent approval rate for all other claims.[27] In a recent lecture, Dr. Paul Cheney stated that, between 1989 and 1993, the largest private insurance carrier in the United States also reported an unprecedented 365 percent increase in claims of CFIDS for men, and a 557 percent increase in claims for women, the highest increase of any disease for this carrier.[28]

One can only assume, given these statistics, that economy plays a large role in the negligence of CFIDS, or many modern conditions. "Being ill is never agreeable," writes Albert Camus in his classic novel, *The Plague*. "An invalid needs small attentions." But for severely ill patients, waiting desperately for research funding that will lead to viable treatments, fiscal neglect can be maddening. As Camus writes: "Think what it must be for a dying man, trapped behind hundreds of walls all sizzling with heat, while the whole population, sitting in cafés or hanging on the telephone, is discussing shipments, bills of lading, discounts!"[29] Indeed, CFIDS patients have also spent years witnessing the benign fiscal and emotional neglect of their suffering, even though they are not living with a terminal disease. They have watched the telethons for other illnesses, the AIDS bike-a-thons, the MS walks, the breast cancer runs, as they have struggled every day to complete the most basic tasks or to secure subpoverty disability wages.

As in the early years of AIDS, perception of the severity and prevalence of CFIDS has simply been skewed by a paucity of public acknowledgment. Without such acknowledgment, the ill tend to stay underground, seek medical help irregularly, and suffer silently. Furthermore, the lack of education in medical schools about CFIDS leads to an untracked demographic. According to the Health Resources and Services Administration (HRSA), only 44 percent of medical schools mention CFIDS in their curricula.[30] Though most people I know with CFIDS have gone to emergency rooms at one time or another, we have all learned that talking about CFIDS generally pushes us further back in the triage queue, so instead we speak the language of acute crisis—*fever, chills, chest pains, dangerously low blood pressure*—too sick and desperate for help to translate the truth to the misinformed. Many patients have been subjected to constant belittling and verbal abuse from doctors who have called them crazy and disbelieved them. One woman on a CFIDS e-mail list group reported that her doctor said she was too "blonde and beautiful" to be so "exhausted"; another responded that her doctor said she was too much of a "beautiful young redhead" to be so ill. A psychosocial clinician and researcher, Patricia Fennell, CSW-R, has found that many CFIDS patients experience "a post-traumatic stress disorder (PTSD)-like syndrome because of the social context in which they are sick."[31] This trauma, she asserts, is caused by abusive and/or ignorant doctors, a negative cultural response, and the overwhelming and continuous grief of remaining sick for a long period of time without relief.

In a climate of medical mystery, many have also tried to find a causal link between CFIDS and preexisting behaviors and personality traits that, in the case of any other illness, would be considered exemplary—blaming patients for having had a strong work ethic (calling them "overachievers"), exercising regularly (being "too driven"), and being empathic (or "too sensitive"). As with much of medicine, this behavior/personality argument has mostly come into play when medicine has failed to find a definitive cause. And because of this, CFIDS patients often internalize medicine's blame-the-victim stance, condemning themselves for every prior excess. I have rarely heard a Lyme disease patient, in contrast, engage in such extensive self-blame about spending too much time hiking in the woods, working in the garden, or visiting relatives in Connecticut.

Ironically, most attributions of personality to CFIDS patients run contrary to current research. While CFIDS is frequently portrayed as a disease of women who cannot handle stress, recent studies suggest that women employ coping methods during stressful events that make them *less* prone to stress-induced illnesses.[32] Some people have even tried to paint a negative profile of CFIDS children and adolescents, insisting that clinical validation of the illness is "an invitation to create invalidism in children."[33] These accusations ignore the quiet magnitude of the problem, or the fact that these children deemed lazy or school-phobic say they miss their active lives. An exhaustive five-year survey of over 333,000 schoolchildren in the United Kingdom in fact found that more than half of the children on long-term sick leave (51 percent) were suffering from ME/CFIDS.[34] The testimonials of such children paint a picture of horribly sick but motivated youth. Fourteen-year-old patient Zac Osgood explained in the *Chicago Tribune:* "Just about every Friday night, all of my friends go out to a party at school or some other kind of activity, while I'm left at home sitting and watching TV—which sounds pretty good, but not for twenty-six straight months." Pictured reading comic books while a technician monitored his heart, Zac seemed inured to the accusations of secondary gain. As if he knew the Make-a-Wish Foundation would never stop by the CFIDS ward, he added, "And with all this there's no reward."[35]

Many people forget that AIDS also struck silently at first, shunned because of an early misnomer (Gay Related Immune Deficiency) that rationalized medical neglect through cultural homophobia. Awareness of the illness, in all countries, remained relative to medical acknowledgment and tracking. *A Small Gathering of Bones* recounts the horror of early AIDS years in Jamaica, when people were dying without a name for their disease, and shame clouded the suffering in mystery. "The telegram didn't specify any particular ailment," the novelist writes, "only that Dale must come."[36] For many years of the AIDS crisis, many also held on to the erroneous belief that AIDS didn't exist in Africa, later finding out that Africa had fallen prey to both the greatest continental scourge of the illness and an even deadlier foe—nonexistent health care access. Now, AIDS is Africa's number one killer, surpassing war as the greatest cause of death. "It is the modern incarnation of Dante's inferno," said UNICEF Deputy Executive Director Stephen Lewis. "Never has Africa faced such a plague."[37] This early mythology of AIDS should have proved to medical humanitarians and scholars that cultural blindness often arises out of poverty, neglect, and unethical medicine. Illness can exist without understanding or definition, but without these two things, it will rarely be helped.

Camus's social commentary and the AIDS crisis both point to a disturbing fact of human nature. Illnesses are rarely legitimated unless they result in death or severe disfigurement. Until these consequences are acutely seen and felt, a mythology follows the ill in their travails. The plague of Camus's novel—which could be any plague—approaches in a similar manner, at first seen, like CFIDS, as but a minor annoyance. "Hitherto people had merely grumbled at a stupid, rather obnoxious visitation," writes Camus. "They now realized that this strange phenomenon, whose scope could not be measured and whose origins escaped detection, had something vaguely menacing about it."[38] The reporter whose notebooks comprise the first early account of the plague, a newcomer to the town, writes from the perspective of an outsider. In this, he is much like the reporters who have written about CFIDS with remote observations, relying on hearsay rather than interviews with patients. The reporter of the plague "seems to make a point of understatement, and at first sight we might almost imagine that [he] had a habit of observing events and people through the wrong end of a telescope."[39]

CFIDS, still a disease diagnosed after a process of elimination, not by a positive blood test, is often likewise defined in the negative, by its inverse, relegated to the gauzy background of pathologies that have frustrated empirical minds. Why else would a *New Yorker* writer describe a hyperefficient subject by saying he "suffers from the opposite of chronic fatigue syndrome?"[40] Would it have been similarly acceptable, queried a friend of mine, to say he suffered from the opposite of a diabetic coma? Of course not. Only in the climate of misinformation could such a dismissive, albeit innocent, description happen. In reality, CFIDS is an extremely complex and debilitating disorder, so mentally and physically disabling that patients have found it nearly impossible to advocate for their own welfare. When syphilis was gravely untreatable, Sir William Osler said, "To understand syphilis is to understand all of medicine." Explains Dr. David Bell, "I cannot think of a better description of CFIDS. Virtually every organ system is involved."[41] Since few doctors "understand all of medicine" these days, CFIDS has been approached from a number of different angles, with specialists entering the labyrinth of illness from all sides. Some researchers think CFIDS is a xenobiotic toxicity disorder; some believe it is a chronically reactivated viral infection (quite possibly involving HHV-6, a virus implicated in both AIDS and MS, though others have theorized about a retrovirus and a "stealth" virus). Others, such as Dr. Jay Goldstein and Dr. Jay Seastrunk, have postulated that CFIDS is the result of a focal brain injury or other brain pathology. Many startling abnormalities have been found in CFIDS patients in almost every bodily system—such as extremely low blood volume, enzyme pathway disruptions, cardiac disturbances, and malfunction of the hypothalamus-pituitary-adrenal axis. Causal theories range from speculation about viruses, bacteria, and mycoplasmas to ideas about the conglomerate effects of multiple chemical exposures to common products (such as pesticides). Two promising lab tests for CFIDS—one involving a urinary marker discovered in Australia that delineates numerous types of CFIDS, another involving an abnormality of an enzyme called RNase L—are pending further research and potential approval. More formative tests show potential: one for an aberrant form of RNA in the bloodstream, and another measuring high urinary levels of a serotonin metabolite called 5-HIAA. Despite the uncertainty of its pathogenesis and etiology, there is no doubt now that CFIDS cases, to the trained eye, are dramatic and severe, existing within strict clinical parameters. The most vague element of the illness has been its etymology.

Though the name of CFIDS is imminently going to change, the history of the name has done irreparable damage. It has already caused many physicians to discount CFIDS altogether, belittle patients, and come to damaging preconceptions. Some forms of alternative medicine, too, have perpetrated a great deal of quackery related to the illness. Many doctors have argued that they simply cannot see anything wrong. But how hard is it—really—to find clinical proof of CFIDS or to debunk ineffective alternative medicine claims? It seems to simply take what Zen masters call a "beginner's mind." Sixteen-year-old Dilnaz Panjwani, for one, made headlines and won top prize at a national Canadian science fair in 1998 when she discovered a statistically significant correlation between low levels of an oxygen-carrying blood enzyme and CFIDS. Because she simply went under the presumption that CFIDS is a difficult and damaging illness that had affected some of her own friends, not a misnamed joke, she was able to uncover a significant abnormality without even going to medical school.[42] Panjwani is also working to develop a blood test for CFIDS, based on her research. In a similar story about young scientists, a fourth-grade science student named Emily Rosa was written up in the *Journal of the American Medical Association* for a simple experiment that debunked a basic premise of a growing field of alternative medicine called therapeutic touch. She proved some twenty-one practitioners of the method were unable to detect a human energy field most of the time, shaking up the methodology of the practice. In its story about Emily, the *Seattle Times* asked a disquieting question: "If a fourth grader can rationally evaluate the difference between valid science and voodoo medicine, why can't more ordinary folks do the same?"[43]

Essentially, what these youth did, and many doctors don't do, is to practice hard science before jumping to conclusions. DePaul University psychology professor Leonard Jason recently proved what patients have known all along: that doctors actually make an unfounded *literary* interpretation of CFIDS patients before employing clinical measures. In a study of 105 Chicago medical students and residents, he found that a scant 22 percent of these trainees believed CFIDS to have a medical cause. The most startling fact of the research, though, is that this presumption correlated directly with the name of the illness, not with actual research or experience with patients. In fact, when alternate names for the illness were used, these students and residents actually changed their prognosis for patients. Jason and his colleagues tested two other names—Florence Nightingale disease (FN), after the famous nurse-activist who suffered from a CFIDS-like illness for many years, and myalgic encepalopathy (ME), a variation of the European term for CFIDS, myalgic encephalomyelitis. Forty-two percent of medical trainees believed FN patients would improve within two years, and 41 percent believed chronic fatigue syndrome patients would improve within two years. In contrast, only 16 percent believed ME patients would improve within two years. The medical-sounding label was enough to make these astute trainees radically alter their perception of the illness.[44] In truth, recovery statistics are even more discouraging. A CDC study followed a number of patients for several years and stated that recovery probability for CFIDS is 48 percent within the first ten years. In this study, however, "recovery" was shakily defined, as *all* of the studied subjects—even those deemed "recovered"—continued to have CFIDS symptoms.[45] A more recent study found that only 4 percent of severe CFIDS patients fully recover, while 39 percent recover partially. This study also found that long-term CFIDS patients are unlikely to turn up with other conditions that would explain their symptoms, and that statistically they may fare worse than those with chronic conditions assumed to have poorer prognoses.[46]

People seem to think that the era of phrenology and medical mysticism and sulfur baths is distant history, but it is not. Where medicine fails, as in the case of CFIDS, health practitioners often make uninformed assumptions, fake knowledge, or offer pseudocures before admitting defeat. Contemporary society has perpetrated a tremendous number of myths about immunity, often grasping onto the persuasive language of quick-fix healing in a desperate attempt to thwart the failings of the body. Certainly, true healing and quackery can happen in both allopathic medicine and alternative medicine. I believe that the scientific method cannot detect some of the more subtle aspects of some healing methods, such as the presence of the subtle energy force Asian healers call *chi.* One time I personally sat in a circle holding hands with seven relative strangers as an astounding—and, I am very convinced, legitimate—Japanese energy healer demonstrated to me how the *chi* of various substances, passed through the bodies of strangers, could cause subtle changes in my own pulse. But I also know that the *Journal of the American Medical Association* printed an analysis of many of the recent studies which supposedly proved the efficacy of alternative medicine methods, finding that every study it looked at "either had a design flaw or showed that alternative practices had an effect that was at or below the level of placebo."[47] This demonstrates to me *not* that alternative medicine is illegitimate, or that allopathic studies are any less likely to have design flaws (they are probably less likely to come under that kind of scrutiny), but simply that patients sometimes must test and retest healing methods themselves, often at their own expense.

And unfortunately, quackery is alive and well, and desperate CFIDS patients are easy targets. In many cases, quacks use pseudomedical language to make bizarre treatments sound more legitimate. Just as doctors can change a prognosis based on language, patients can be sucked into the seductive lingo of quacks. One feverish and homebound day, I even found myself strangely beguiled by an article about the resurgence of an ancient method of "healing," one its proponents say is designed to increase blood flow to the brain by recreating the kind of stronger brain pulse that babies —with softer skulls—have. CFIDS patients, on SPECT scans, are shown to have decreased blood flow to the brain.[48] So, had this article not been about the revived practice of trepanation, or drilling a hole in the skull to release intercranial pressure, I could have been persuaded by its medical lingo that talked about increased "brain blood volume" and purported to alleviate some of the symptoms I know I have. As it is, I am not so gullible, desperate, or masochistic. But if it had been about craniosacral massage, I might have tried it. And when medical schools do not teach about an illness, and a drill is cheaper than a Medicare co-payment, how do we define our experts? As I said before, language and stories—along with economy, assumption, and desperation—often dictate the treatment of the sick.[49]

It is often much harder to separate clinical perversity and exploitation from legitimate medicine than one might think, especially when medical terminology slips through the sieve of the addled CFIDS brain. Although I was never in danger of resorting to home electric drill therapy, I have done things that—at certain times and places in history—might have seemed suspect, such as allowing a Chinese doctor to decorate my body with needles along energy meridians, or paying a chiropractor to crack my spine. Because I am interested in modern quackery and phenomenology, I also read more about the barbaric and disturbing descriptions of those trepanning their skulls. Ironically, the day after I read these accounts, a CFIDS patient posted to a clinically astute CFIDS e-mail list group I am on. She discovered, seven years into her struggle with CFIDS, that she also suffered from a brain stem and spinal cord compression disorder called Arnold-Chiari malformation—a condition that creates symptoms with much CFIDS diagnostic overlap and, according to neurosurgeons such as Dr. Dan Heffetz, may contribute to the debility of a percentage of CFIDS patients.[50] After corrective surgery by a neurosurgeon that involved "cutting away the back of her skull, decompressing the brain, removing the top vertebrae and sewing a graft in place to hold the brain in position," she described herself as being "completely normal and healthy." I couldn't help but notice how much the language of her surgery resembled that of the tripped-out trepanation society, and in fact resembled even more closely the depictions of trepanation doctors in ancient times. The point is that discussions about bone saws, trepans, brain perfusion, and cervical spine abnormalities can borrow from a similar language. Healing has always been a faddish art form, strongly influenced by social and linguistic trends. Patients sit in the middle of this dilution of terminology, trying to sort out quackery from true healing.

Semantics should not hold up the treatment of a group of people who are clearly suffering, but unfortunately—with CFIDS—they have.

As Camus writes about the plague, "Most people were chiefly aware of what ruffled the normal tenor of their lives or affected their interests. They were worried and irritated—but these are not feelings with which to confront plague."[51] Truly, the derisive attitude of the public, the media, the government, and most doctors has been palpable to the CFIDS population, but these are not feelings with which to confront a serious epidemic. A name should not prevent millions of people worldwide from attaining care for very clear, very horrific, suffering. Similarly, in Camus's plague, the town officials argue whether or not to call it "plague" as people go on suffering and dying. The secrecy over the name and the precautionary measures people are asked to take provoke mass suspicion. But one doctor, a compassionate soul who actually has one-on-one contact with patients, says, "You're stating the problem wrongly. It's not a question of the term I use; it's a question of time."[52]

Indeed, for the months and years of imprisonment that CFIDS thrusts upon its victims, made up of unrelenting symptomatology, it is a question of time. And much time has passed already with very little progress. There are no cures for CFIDS, and no drugs specifically approved by the FDA to treat CFIDS. The CDC is slowly restoring the funds stolen from CFIDS accounts—necessary funds that, by the auditor's own record, were actually used to "balance the books at the end of each fiscal year." This procedure was so corrupt that the agency is beginning to take corrective actions that it describes as "the most far-reaching in the half-century history of the CDC."[53] Still, research is horribly underfunded and thus tediously slow. One hopeful drug called Ampligen, tested on CFIDS patients by default, held up for years in bureaucracy, still controversial because of its adverse reactions, is pending final FDA approval. But CFIDS patients tread in precarious waters. Because of negative publicity questioning the legitimacy of CFIDS, the company that makes Ampligen almost folded when its stock dropped, and patients fear that more bad press will make it (or other drugs) unavailable to patients. Currently, many are desperate for Ampligen, willing to shell out anywhere from $15,000 to $40,000 a year on the drug company's cost-recovery program if they are lucky enough to be one of the handful on the approved list. It is hard for anyone to be patient after months and years in bed.

Although many have played a role in the neglect of the CFIDS epidemic, this is not a book about naming scapegoats. I hope it will instead allow people to question their foundational knowledge of medicine, healing, and disability. The CFIDS epidemic speaks to many critical issues of this era. If household insecticides are essentially "diluted forms of chemical warfare agents," as Gary Null asserts (a provocative but true statement, as pesticides were originally created in World War II as nerve gas weapons), and diagnosis is, as Susan Griffin writes, a process of democracy, I hope *Stricken* will help people to search for a more ethical government of the body, the environment, and medicine itself.

The public conception of CFIDS is still changing. At the time of this writing, CFIDS actually goes by many names. Chronic fatigue syndrome (CFS), chronic fatigue immune dysfunction syndrome (CFIDS), and myalgic encephalomyelitis (ME) are the most common, though strong evidence suggests that Gulf War syndrome (GWS) is a form of CFIDS[54] (the Surgeon General of the Army and the CDC have both admitted that GWS is a CFIDS-like disorder).[55] Fibromyalgia and multiple chemical sensitivities (MCS) are two conditions that also often overlap, but are not synonymous, with CFIDS. *Stricken* includes those who are incarcerated in the minimum security of their own bedrooms, and also those in the familial and political arena. Because of the shifting platform of symptomatology and naming, I have drawn upon the longstanding tradition of poets as the alchemists of language to convey some of the more amorphous aspects of the illness experience. I have also included pieces that have a call to revolution tenor, some that deconstruct volatile political issues of this hidden epidemic, and others that are highly personal. As bedroom practices intersect with politics even at the presidential level, I think it's time for this bedridden and semihomebound underground to have an eloquent, accurate, and sometimes incendiary public voice.

NOTES

1. Wallich, Paul. "Senile Words." *Scientific American,* June 1996, pp. 26-28.

2. Komaroff, Anthony L., Richard B. Schwartz, Basem M. Garada, Harold M. Tice, Marcy Gleit, Ferenc A. Jolesz, and B. Leonard Holman. "SPECT Imaging of the Brain: Comparison of Findings in Patients with Chronic Fatigue Syndrome, AIDS

Dementia Complex, and Major Unipolar Depression." *American Journal of Roentgenology, 162,* April 1994, pp. 943-951.

3. Johnson, Hillary. *Osler's Web.* New York: Crown Publishers, 1996, pp. 78-80.

4. Cheney, Paul. From a lecture sponsored by the Greater Philadelphia CFIDS Alliance titled "A CFIDS Symposium: Critical Issues." Temple University, November 1998.

5. Johnson, *Osler's Web,* p. 130.

6. "Writing May Ease Symptoms." *The CFIDS Chronicle,* May/June 1999, p. 13.

7. Kenney, K. Kimberly. "Wichita Study Reveals Much About Who Has CFIDS." *The CFIDS Chronicle,* November/December 1998, p. 25.

8. Knox, Richard A. "Funding for Chronic Fatigue Diverted, Report Says." *The Boston Globe,* May 16, 1999.

9. From a letter written by Chairman Marc Iverson of the CFIDS Association of America to its members, dated June 17, 1999.

10. Mitchell, Alison. "Starr Has Hired Ex-Federal Agents in Investigation of Clinton." *The New York Times,* October 29, 1998, p. A25.

11. CNN/Time. "Sick and Tired." Aired on television October 24, 1999. (Transcript at CNN Web site: <http://cnn.com/transcripts/9910/24/impc.00.html>.)

12. Ouellette, Dan. "A Piano Genius Battles Back: Keith Jarrett Emerges from Long Bout of Chronic Fatigue to Perform Tonight." Sunday Datebook, *San Francisco Chronicle,* February 28, 1999, p. 37.

13. AIDS specialist Dr. Mark Loveless testified at a May 12, 1995, congressional briefing sponsored by Illinois Congressman John Porter and Nevada Senator Harry Reid.

14. Johnson, *Osler's Web,* p. 364.

15. Anderson J.S. and C.E. Ferrans. "The Quality of Life of Persons with Chronic Fatigue Syndrome." *Journal of Nervous and Mental Disorders, 185*(6), June 1997, pp. 359-367. Jason, Leonard A., Renée R. Taylor, Cara L. Kennedy, Sharon Song, Danielle Johnson, and Carrie J. Curie. "Shattering the Myths: Recommendations from a Community-Based Study of CFS." *The CFS Research Review, 1*(1), Winter 2000, p. 5.

16. Leonard Jason, interviewed by Elizabeth "Ebus" Estes-Cooper on WJBC Radio, Bloomington, IL, May 12, 2000.

17. Bell, David. "Tired All the Time: A Chat with Dr. David Bell." *CFIDS and Fibromyalgia Healthwatch,* Spring 1999 Edition, p. 14.

18. CNN/Time, "Sick and Tired."

19. Goodman, Ellen. "The Babes of Summer: A Women's Movement if There Ever Was One." *The Boston Globe,* July 15, 1999, p. A25.

20. Search of *The New York Times* Web site <www.nyt.com> archives conducted on July 9, 1999. I eliminated duplicate articles in my research on "chronic fatigue syndrome," then read each article to make sure it contained "chronic fatigue syndrome" as a sequence, not as three separate words in the article. I did not read all the articles on the other diseases I mentioned, simply cited the number the search engine gave me and mentioned interesting titles.

21. Williams, Thomas D. "Chronic Fatigue Research Funds Were Diverted." *The Hartford Courant,* June 3, 1999, p. A10.

22. Carpman, Vicki. "San Francisco Prevalence Study Alters CFS Profile." *The CFIDS Chronicle,* Winter 1997, p. 82.

23. Jason, Leonard A., Judith A. Richman, Alfred W. Rademaker, Karen M. Jordan, Audrius V. Plioplys, Renée R. Taylor, William McCready, Cheng-Fang Huang, and Sigita Plioplys. "A Community-Based Study of Chronic Fatigue Syndrome." *Archives of Internal Medicine, 159* (18), October 11, 1999, pp. 2129-2137.

24. Bell, David S. *The Doctor's Guide to Chronic Fatigue Syndrome.* New York: Addison-Wesley Publishing, 1995, p. 14.

25. Johnson, *Osler's Web,* p. 363.

26. Ibid., p. 143.

27. Kenney, K. Kimberly. "Social Security Disability: Protecting Access for PWCs." *The CFIDS Chronicle,* Summer 1996, p. 40.

28. Cheney, Paul. Lecture. The Third International Congress of Bioenergetic Medicine, Orlando, Florida, February 6, 1999.

29. Camus, Albert. *The Plague.* Translated by Stuart Gilbert. New York: Vintage Books, 1991, p. 5.

30. "Medical Students Learn About CFIDS." *The CFIDS Chronicle,* Winter 1997, p. 5.

31. Carpman, Vicki L. "Keynote Address: Patricia A. Fennell, CSW-R." *The CFIDS Chronicle,* Fall 1995, p. 24.

32. Jablon, Robert. "Stress May Help Women Live Healthier." The Associated Press Newswire, May 19, 2000.

33. Showalter, Elaine. *Hystories: Hysterical Epidemics and Modern Media.* New York: Columbia University Press, 1997, p. 132.

34. Dowsett, Elizabeth and Jane Colby. "Long Term Sickness Absence Due to ME/CFS in Schools." *Journal of Chronic Fatigue Syndrome, 3*(2), 1997, pp. 29-42.

35. Osgood, Charles. "Meet Zac: He's Really Sick of Being Tired." *Chicago Tribune Magazine,* November 15, 1998, p. 27.

36. Powell, Patricia. *A Small Gathering of Bones.* Oxford: Heinemann, 1994, p. 81.

37. Mwangi, George. "AIDS Overtakes War As African Killer." The Associated Press Syndicated News Service, July 21, 1999.

38. Camus, *The Plague,* p. 16.

39. Ibid., p. 24.

40. Owen, David. "The Sultan of Stuff." *The New Yorker,* July 19, 1999, p. 54.

41. Bell, *The Doctor's Guide to Chronic Fatigue Syndrome,* p. 13.

42. "Canadian Teen Finds Correlation with Blood Enzyme." *The CFIDS Chronicle,* July/August 1998, p. 11.

43. "Fourth-Grade Science." *The Seattle Times,* April 4, 1998, p. A13.

44. Jason, Leonard A., Renée R. Taylor, Sigita Plioplys, and Zuzanna Stepanek. "Study Compares Medical Trainees' Reactions to Three Names for CFS." *The CFIDS Chronicle,* July/August 1999, p. 18. Also: "New Chronic Fatigue Study

Fuels Debate on Name Change; DePaul Professor Says Biological Name Taken More Seriously." *PR Newswire,* August 26, 1999. <http://www.prnewswire.com>.

45. Reyes, Michele, James G. Dobbins, Rosane Nisenbaum, Nazerah S. Subedar, Bonnie Randall, and William C. Reeves. "Chronic Fatigue Syndrome Progression and Self-Defined Recovery: Evidence from CDC Surveillance System." *Journal of Chronic Fatigue Syndrome, 5*(1), 1999, pp. 17-27.

46. Hill, Nancy F., Lana A. Tiersky, Vanessa R. Scavalla, Marc Lavietes, and Benjamin H. Natelson. "National History of Severe Chronic Fatigue Syndrome." *Archives of Physical Medicine and Rehabilitation, 80,* September 1999, pp. 1090-1094.

47. Stoler, David Andrew. "Alternative Medicine: Miracle Cure or Malpractice?" *The Providence Phoenix,* June 25, 1999, p. 10.

48. Richardson, John and Durval Campos Costa. "Relationship Between SPECT Scans and Buspirone Tests in Patients with ME/CFS." *The Journal of Chronic Fatigue Syndrome, 4*(3), 1998, pp. 22-33.

49. Bowen, Joh. "The Hole Thing." *The Providence Phoenix,* June 4, 1999, p. 14.

50. "Can Spinal Surgery Really Help?" *The CFIDS Chronicle,* November/December 1999, p. 22.

51. Camus, *The Plague,* p. 78.

52. Ibid., p. 50.

53. Brehio, Renee. "CDC Admits Wrongdoing." *The CFIDS Chronicle,* September/October 1999, pp. 6-7.

54. Nicolson, Garth L. "Chronic Fatigue Illness and Operation Desert Storm." *Journal of Occupational and Environmental Medicine, 38*(1), January 1996, p. 14; Hoh, David. "Gulf War Syndrome linked to CFIDS: Symptoms Match, CDC Reports." *The CFIDS Chronicle,* Summer 1997, p. 19.

55. "Gulf War Syndrome, CFIDS Link Gains More Recognition." *The CFIDS Chronicle,* September/October 1999, p. 21.

PART I:
DOUBT AND DIAGNOSIS

Chapter 1

Encounters with the Invisible

Dorothy Wall

You would think we'd be used to the invisible in this information age with its reliance on electronic data and cyberspace and hyperreality. Used to the fact that we depend on things we can't see, that don't even exist except as a concept, a social agreement held by people we've never met or heard of.

But in fact, we're as distrustful, as apprehensive, as unbelieving of the invisible as if we still equated it with spirits, ethers, and ghouls. For all our New Age mantras about inner spirit and higher power, we're still a decidedly practical people and if someone is ill we want proof. A test, a diagnosis. Evidence.

As a person with chronic fatigue immune dysfunction syndrome (CFIDS), I don't have much to offer. My body is intact. I have no crusty blood, no sour-smelling secretions, seeping wounds, swollen flesh. No unsightly scars, no bandages, tubes, bruises. No suspicious blood tests or X rays, no growths. My injuries are invisible, subtle, in neurons, enzymes, cytokines, the intricate inner circuitry of the body that still eludes concise theories, that requires scientific minds to make a leap of faith, to become, as it were, believers.

When I first dragged myself into the doctor's office in 1978 with a high fever, the attending physician took one look at my jaundiced skin, palpated my swollen liver, drew blood, and came back with an instant diagnosis: mononucleosis. I was a doctor's delight: clear symptoms, easy conclusion. Even more gratifying, the flesh above my eyelids was swollen, a symptom of mono recorded in medical books but occurring so rarely that the doctor, in his fifties, had never seen it and seemed inordinately pleased that I had provided him simultaneously with this rare sighting and confirmation of the solidity and reliability of his medical training.

But at that point, I was only beginning my venture into the land of illness. A year and a half later, with the onset of CFIDS, the textbook neatness of my mononucleosis symptoms would degenerate into the perplexing array of complaints no textbook could explain: recurring brain fog, sinus pressure, sore throat, fatigue, yet all blood tests normal. I have an enduring picture of one doctor after another peering at me with that poker face that means they're madly trying to compute the subtext: Was I a malingerer? Did I evidence emotional imbalance? Was I having family problems? This illness would confound rather than confirm their training, leaving me in the absurd position of having to insist, explain, educate, be lucid, believable, convincing, all while so weak and confused and out-of-it that I could hardly speak.

"Why are you so weak?" asked the doctor who saw me in 1995 upon my return from a business trip to New York. I knew I was very ill, but I didn't yet know that my trip had triggered a severe exacerbation of the CFIDS that had waxed and waned over the previous fifteen years.

In the way of HMOs, where a different doctor appears each time you're there—revolving-door doctors, or roulette doctors, I call them—this doctor was a woman I'd never seen before. I was lying on the exam table in a stupor of exhaustion. My body felt pressed against the vinyl as if I were on a planet with two Gs. From his chair against the wall, my partner Bill had explained when she came into the room that I had chronic fatigue syndrome and a sinus infection and had just returned Friday from New York quite ill.

By Sunday night my sinus infection was so intense I felt as if someone had poured concrete down my face, through my cranium, neck, shoulders, and halfway down my back. I needed more antibiotics—the doctor I had seen in New York had given me only a three-day supply. That Monday morning Bill had driven me to the medical center, dropped me at the curb, then gone to park. It was only twenty yards to the foyer, but once inside I was astounded at the exhaustion I felt, wobbly legged and rocky, as if I'd just stepped off a boat. The comings and goings of people around me seemed distant and confusing. It occurred to me I might not make it to the doctor's office on the third floor and I looked around for a wheelchair and some assistance. I didn't see anything. It seemed easier just to get myself upstairs.

I made it to the elevator, stunned by the weakness in my legs, the pressure in my chest, as if I had to push against tightly stretched canvas to breathe. On the third floor I saw the length of hallway ahead and sagged. I was afraid I might collapse on the floor right there. I thought maybe I should. Bill would find me and bring a wheelchair. Dazed, I stumbled forward in a robotic, Frankenstein lurch, arms out for balance, willing myself to put one foot in front of the other down that hallway. A woman ahead of me, alarmed, leaped to hold open the heavy glass door. I slid to a chair in the waiting room. When Bill came he brought me a wheelchair.

The doctor stood on the other side of the exam room, my chart in front of her, and eyed me clinically, clearly suspicious of the wheelchair crowding the small cubicle. She read the notations on my chart. Blood pressure normal. Temperature 99.3. Nothing unusual. Slight sore throat, chest clear. She took my blood pressure again, standing up and lying down. Normal. Took my pulse lying down, then had me stand and laid her fingers on my wrist again. Ah. My pulse raced from the simple exertion of standing.

This gave me a tiny iota of credibility. This was measurable, tangible. But it wasn't enough. Rounding up the usual suspects, she wanted me tested for anemia, thyroid, diabetes. Weakly, I shook my head. I knew all blood tests would come back normal, as they had throughout this illness. I could no more explain to her the years of exhaustion, brain fog, chronic sore throat, the catastrophic collapse I had just endured in New York trying to finish research for a book, than I could have given a speech in a lecture hall. I lay back down on the crinkly paper of the exam table.

There are many kinds of invisibility, and CFIDS is layered with them. The most striking is that despite a person's symptoms and complaints (like most people with CFIDS, I've developed an impressive array: fatigue, low-grade fever, night sweats, swollen lymph nodes, sore throat, mouth sores, nausea, sinus pain, joint and muscle aches, musculoskeletal tenderness, headache, earache, muscle weakness, sleep disturbance, brain fog, confusion, light and sound sensitivity), the body, amazingly, offers up no firm evidence of a microbial pathogen. The cause of this illness remains unknown, shrouded in mystery and controversy.

A virus is the main suspect, but viruses come in all types and guises and are masters of evasion. They can hide, mutate, combine, and eerily escape detection. We suspect their presence based on the damage they do, the symptoms they produce, the antibodies produced in response to their presence, but we often never see them. There has been much focus on a retrovirus as the cause, but the research supporting this theory remains mired in controversy. Many researchers now believe no single agent is responsible for CFIDS, that the illness is in fact a cluster of illnesses, too complex to be explained by a single pathogen. Genetic, environmental, and disease processes may all be implicated to create a complex illness picture.

One researcher, pathologist John Martin, has hypothesized that CFIDS is caused by a "stealth" virus, a DNA virus that infects the brain and may play a part in a number of illnesses, including atypical encephalopathies and subacute brain disease. The image of stealth is fitting for an illness whose causative agent slides under the radar of our available instrumentation.

If the illness remains elusive, so do its effects. CFIDS is an invisible disability. You can be profoundly ill and still look fine. Because I first became ill in 1980, before anything was known about CFIDS, I spent many years going through life exhausted but keeping up appearances. It was easy to do. No doctor believed I was ill. I didn't look ill. And I didn't want to think of myself as ill. The exhaustion, brain fog, and recurring sore throat that kept a steady backbeat to my life as a single mother, teacher, and writing consultant were mostly private facts of life.

Even after CFIDS was acknowledged by the Centers for Disease Control in 1988, physicians remained either suspicious or uncomprehending of my complaints. Once I was seeing my internist, an amiable man who knew I had CFIDS, for a routine checkup. At that time I was well enough to get out for three or four hours in the midday. During those precious hours I saw writing clients, ran errands, scheduled appointments.

This doctor was cheerfully palpating my breasts for lumps, chatting away. He mentioned he had just seen the musical *Cats,* and recommended I go see it. It's not easy to be assertive while you're lying on your back in a blue paper gown. I waited until he completed the exam, pulled myself up with as much dignity as possible while clutching the flaps of my paper vest, and looked him in the eye. "Doctor, I'm not able to go to plays in the evening. I have CFIDS. My day is basically over by late afternoon."

"Oh," he beamed. "You look fine to me."

The woefully inadequate understanding this otherwise fine doctor had of CFIDS is widespread, and it's not just because those with CFIDS look suspiciously well. There exists in the medical community of doctors, scientists, and bureaucrats a pervasive bias that has kept this illness from legitimacy and recognition. Hillary Johnson's revealing book *Osler's Web: Inside the Labyrinth of the Chronic Fatigue Syndrome Epidemic* chronicles how the Centers for Disease Control and the National Institutes of Health resisted legitimizing this illness, how the politics of research funding prevented investigation, and how the physicians who did take CFIDS seriously were ridiculed and ostracized. She writes compellingly of the way "the bias of federal scientists and their bureaucratic machinations compounded to the erase the epidemic from public view."[1]

In the early 1990s the CDC estimated the number of people with CFIDS to be between 2 and 10 per 100,000, a figure that subsequently came under fire from patient advocacy groups. In part because of their pressure, in 1998 the CDC conducted a prevalence study in Wichita, Kansas, and surrounding Sedgwick County, an area demographically similar to the entire United States.

Unlike the previous study, which relied on doctors to report the disease (the very doctors who often discount or fail to recognize this illness), the researchers in Wichita called one quarter of the population, asked questions about fatigue, then evaluated in a clinic those who had CFIDS-like symptoms to determine if they did in fact have CFIDS. When looking at an entire community rather than only those people with access to health care and persistence in obtaining a diagnosis, the researchers concluded that a staggering 183 people per 100,000 have CFIDS, almost twenty times the CDC's highest original estimate.[2] Subsequently, Dr. Leonard Jason's 1999 community-based study in Chicago, Illinois, among a more ethnically diverse population, revealed a prevalence rate of 422 per 100,000, which translates to roughly 800,000 adults in the United States with CFIDS.[3]

Besides revealing CFIDS as a major public health problem, the Wichita and Chicago studies paint an astounding picture of an invisible community, struggling to maintain lives without the benefit of diagnosis, validation, medical support, or treatment.

This public erasure is often reenacted within the self as a self-erasure, a silence about illness. In the face of disbelief and ignorance you have to be brazen to be visible, to be out about your illness. And the enervating fatigue of illness doesn't make you feel brazen. People with CFIDS often find it easier to go incognito, or to tell the people in their lives of their illness on a need-to-know basis, rather than face the misunderstandings, projections, and well-meaning suggestions of others with little or no knowledge of this illness. When I walked through my day behind a filmy screen of exhaustion, the last thing I wanted was for someone to tell me of the latest cure for fatigue they'd heard of from their neighbor's cousin's boyfriend. "Passing" as a well person becomes an act of self-preservation, allowing dignity, control, and a chance to maintain a preillness identity, often vital to one's sense of self. It also increases the already profound invisibility of this illness.

CFIDS' invisibility is further contoured by language, or rather, its lack. Without an adequate medical understanding, there's no accepted medical language to identify CFIDS and bring it into view. The name itself, chronic fatigue syndrome, basically translates: a bunch of symptoms no one understands. I can't toss off a succinct, scary-sounding name for this illness, a tidy, impressive cause. Once when I called the advice nurse at my HMO to get an appointment, so weak I could barely talk, she said to me, "I heard it's not really an illness. What do you think?"

Ironically, medical language works to narrow and flatten the complex, personal encounter with illness, reducing a lived experience to notations on physiological and biochemical states. To say I have brain stem perfusion doesn't describe the painful effort of trying to make a thought connect through a brain that feels like a block of wood, or the disorientation of being unable to string together a sequence of actions: put on dark glasses, find keys, lock door. To talk about decreased plasma corticosterone and impaired responsiveness of the hypothalamic-pituitary-adrenal axis doesn't capture the anger, frustration, or sense of loss that an ill person daily feels when unable even to drive to the market or prepare a simple meal.

Yet medical language, for all its inadequacy, assuages skeptical minds. It provides legitimacy to a person's complaints and symptoms, and justifies those weeks and months in bed. Words have the power, like superstitions, to redeem, to brand, to conjure belief and disbelief. If I say I have myalgic encephalomyelitis (ME), the name for CFIDS used in England and many other countries (myalgic means muscle pain, encephalomyelitis means inflammation of the brain), people respond very differently than if I say I have chronic fatigue syndrome. ME carries scientific weight; it sounds substantive.

In fact, there has been a raging debate within the CFIDS community about the name chronic fatigue syndrome, between those who feel it trivializes the illness and want to change it, and those who feel that despite its limitations, the name has gained some public recognition and should be maintained. It's expected that a new name will be chosen soon. The name was originally selected by CDC investigator Gary Holmes and associates in 1988 because it was purely descriptive, free of "a specific association with any known etiologic agent."[4] Given the lack of understanding of the illness, the choice seemed reasonable. Unfortunately, unanchored to a specific disease process, the name leaves a potent void, inviting an imaginative array of innocent misconceptions (have you checked for food allergies?) and profound prejudices (it's an emotional illness), and rendering the illness itself remote, misty, unseen.

Without a medical language, it's hard to develop a personal language, a language to share our experience. If someone has cancer, we know what follows: surgery, chemotherapy, radiation, hair loss, weakness, nausea. We know what these words mean. They sink in with sharp, terrifying recognition. If I tell someone I have chronic fatigue syndrome, they're likely to say, "Yeah, I'm tired all the time too." Or, "A friend of mine had that, but I think she was depressed." Those of us with CFIDS find ourselves developing our own language ("I feel episody," "I'm fogged out"), a language that operates as a private code among the ill rather than a source of connection with the well.

Add to that the literal invisibility of the person acutely ill with CFIDS, in bed, out of sight. As a writer I've always been intrigued with the invisible. Writers are supposed to believe in the ineffable. We struggle to hoist this elusive dimension into view through language. But now I myself had become the invisible thing.

I went home from the doctor that day in the fall of 1995, clutching my vial of antibiotics, and fell into bed for three months. It would be nine months before I could walk to the corner and back, a year and a half before I could walk into the doctor's office without a wheelchair. I was shut in, my public presence gone. No more teaching, conferences, meetings. I had become a late-twentieth-century Emily Dickinson imitator, my life enclosed, the world viewed through a bedroom window. The edges of pine tree and maple framed my world. Hummingbirds darted past, a breeze, a sling of vaporous clouds, bringing to life this still etching I observed day after day.

Ironically, my disappearance, my erasure from public life, was my body's way of demanding to be seen. The whirls and spurts of hormones, lymphocyte surges, macrophage assaults, were no longer subtle, hidden affairs. They were flagrant, in fevers, rashes, sores and sweats, incapacitating fatigue. My body's protest against the pressures of my active life became impossible to discount.

I was the one who now saw my illness more clearly. In this quiet, reclusive place, away from hustle and busyness, I could see my body for what it was, in struggle with its inner imbalances, needing extra tending and care. Though I had known I had limits, even I had been fooled by the invisibility of this illness into thinking I could keep soldiering on. I couldn't. This seeing, this acknowledgment, was what would open the door to healing and bring me back to the world.

NOTES

1. Johnson, Hillary. *Osler's Web.* New York: Crown Publishers, 1996, p. 564.

2. Kenney, K. Kimberly. "Wichita Study Reveals Much About Who Has CFIDS." *The CFIDS Chronicle,* November/December 1998, p. 25.

3. Jason, Leonard A., Judith A. Richman, Alfred W. Rademaker, Karen M. Jordan, Audrius V. Plioplys, Renée R. Taylor, William McCready, Cheng-Fang Huang, and Sigita Plioplys. "A Community-Based Study of Chronic Fatigue Syndrome." *Archives of Internal Medicine, 159* (18), October 11, 1999, pp. 2129-2137.

4. Johnson, *Osler's Web,* p. 231.

Chapter 2

From *What Her Body Thought: A Journey into the Shadows*

Susan Griffin

FROM "SUSTENANCE"

In the first decade after CFIDS was identified, a prejudicial and nearly tautological reasoning was applied to the illness, as if its existence could be explained away. The medical establishment drew a profile of the person most likely to come down with the disease. A mature woman, professional, upper middle class, white, and overly ambitious, she did not know how to rest, and this is why she was fatigued. The description recalls those tracts from nineteenth-century medicine warning that higher education could damage a woman's ovaries. Both theories have a subtext, the idea that women ought to stay at home. And I can hear another suggestion in the thought, the subtle warning that feminism undermines the feminine body.

The image of CFIDS as a white middle-class women's disease is hard to live down. It lingers in the public mind, so that people are still surprised to learn that there are children, African-American, Hispanic, Asian men and women of all classes and ages who have the disease. The profile turns out to be wrong. The error occurred because of the way the statistics were gathered. Doctors were asked to report the number of patients they had diagnosed with CFIDS. Yet such a diagnosis is available only to those with the financial means to pay for a battery of tests or, encountering the earlier bias of the medical establishment, to go from doctor to doctor, searching for one who accepts the reality of the illness.

But the story takes an even grimmer turn. Instead of searching for a virus, supporting extensive laboratory tests, or even conducting epidemiological studies aimed at finding environmental triggers, the National Institutes of Health focused on a single study, one that searched for psychological causes. Stephen Straus, who initiated the study, announced its results to the media. His data showed, he claimed, that a large number of patients with CFIDS he studied had some history of mental disturbance. His statements made an indelible impression in the press. Even today, after clear and ample evidence of the physical etiology of the illness, every once in a while a celebrity doctor still appears on my local television station and, with his boyish good looks and charming manner, casually tells his audience that the disease I have is largely the effect of neurosis.

Yet just like the profile, the study too was wrong. Violating the most basic procedure of statistical science, Straus had used no control group. When another statistician supplied one, comparing the study of Straus's patients to a corresponding group without the illness, he found the rate of mental illness in both groups to be the same.

It is difficult to describe the effect of being told you are not really ill when you are. The disjuncture between private experience and public image is so severe, you can easily become obsessed with establishing the truth. The degree of discomfort felt so intensely in body and soul at such a fracture could itself be a subject for psychosomatic medicine. As certainly as a kind of epiphany is achieved with naming, a shock of recognition that can be physically felt, so also an equally intense and negative shock is experienced with misnaming. It is a sinking feeling, something like missing a train for a journey that is not at all casual. You are left hanging. Disoriented. Strangely lonely. Though this will not be a peaceful solitude. You will be followed into your privacy by phantoms of rejection and even ridicule for what your body continues to know. The sound of these phantoms may be inaudible, but it will be distracting enough to erase your own voice, to quell any attempt to articulate even for yourself what it is you experience. And this is a serious loss because it is this voice, the intelligent and observing companion to feeling, that dignifies even the worst misery.

FROM "DEMOCRACY"

If at times all of us feel disempowered in a world run by giant corporations and governments increasingly beyond the reach of the people, the sense of disempowerment increases exponentially when you are ill. It is not just the frailty of illness that weakens you, though physical weakness certainly deepens the feeling. To be a patient in the labyrinth of modern medicine is to become disenfranchised at an almost primal level. Regarding your own body, it will seem like almost any other opinion carries more weight than your own. As you are told what in the range of your complaints has meaning and what has none, or even at times what you ought to be feeling, your own knowledge weakens.

The most common, seemingly innocuous procedures of medicine serve to strip a patient, not only of dignity, but also of the capacity for autonomous judgment. Asked to somehow describe complex symptoms in the small boxes of an admitting form and to answer yes or no to questions for which only a far more nuanced response would be truthful; made to repeat your complaint several times over, once to a receptionist, once to an aide, once again to a nurse, many of whom seem vaguely disinterested and none of whom are allowed to tell you anything about your condition. Dressed in a gown that leaves you exposed and cold, even if you have a flu or bronchitis or pneumonia. This must have been what it was like to wait at court for an audience.

The disenfranchisement only continues in the process of diagnosis. But here the problem is not just with medical procedure. Trying to express what you feel in your body, you will confront a paucity of words. European languages lack the vocabulary you need to describe physical sensations with any precision, especially symptoms that are painful or uncomfortable. This alone will leave you fumbling in a fog of vague impressions, certain that what you feel remains unnamed. And then there is the hierarchic order of medicine, the doctor often acting more like a lawyer with quick and pointed questions. Some of his questions may baffle you. Others are easy. But still your efforts to describe what you feel will all too frequently be frustrated by an invisible veil of preconceptions, ideas in medical books, maps of the body, prejudices regarding who gets which disease and why, who should or should not be believed. And all along you suspect that while you labor to paint a portrait of a territory your doctor has never experienced in his own body, he will weigh laboratory results far more heavily than your testimony.

When what you know is ignored, the dismissal can be psychologically painful. But the invalidation of the patient's knowledge can also have disastrous effects on your health. It happened to a friend recently, a middle-aged woman just a few years older than I. For a full year she complained to her doctor about a pain in her leg that steadily worsened. When she would tell him she was worried, time and again he assured her that the pain was not caused by anything serious. He diagnosed sciatica at first. And then when the physical therapy he ordered did not help, he wrote her a prescription for Valium. Finally, as she became increasingly disabled, it was difficult for her to climb up onto his examining table. But rather than noting the growing severity of her condition, he told her to hurry up. "There are people who are *really* sick who need to be seen today," he said. It would be months before she finally received the right diagnosis, this time from a young doctor on the emergency ward who could feel the problem with his hands. A malignant tumor had eaten through her femur.

There are many doctors who listen more closely and with greater compassion. Yet within a system that diminishes the significance of a patient's testimony, everyone tends to err in the direction of ignorance. Surprisingly, it is physical experience itself that is ignored. Even with the most sensitive practitioners, you will seldom be asked to give full witness to the life of your body. And because on an unspoken level of mind, you learn how to treat yourself from the way that you are treated by others, especially authority figures, the effect of this narrow focus can be to limit the range of your own attention. Many times after visiting a doctor who did not listen well, I have found myself turning away from the habit of awareness, trying to ignore what I feel myself. The eventual effect, if you are in pain or discomfort, can be a subtle resignation, the sense that nothing could or perhaps should be done to help you.

The resignation is similar to the resignation the working poor will sometimes feel. As if the hard circumstances of their lives were inevitable somehow. Which is also how society often makes them feel. The similarity is perhaps understandable if only because, just as stories are the stuff of democracy, economy is an extension of the body. Who shall prosper, who shall not, who shall have pleasure, who shall be deprived, even, at times, who shall live and who shall die. You will certainly feel economy as continuous with your own body if you are fighting to survive.

And the circumstances of poverty and medical neglect share this too, something I have felt just underneath my own resignation: the sense that my body was somehow at fault not only for being ill, but also for having an untreatable or even unnamed condition, for failing, in fact, to fit into the profile of what is an abstract body, the one that medicine creates from studies and statistics.

Dissociated, kinesthetically akimbo, as if pasted together from instructions written in a foreign language, strangely uncoordinated, this Frankensteinian body can at best provide only a distorted mirror of experience. When my doctor, who was intuitively astute, offered the diagnosis of an immune disorder to me, because she had not experienced the illness herself, her only recourse was to read a list of symptoms that had come down, like pronouncements from Sinai, from the Centers for Disease Control. But I could not recognize my own condition in this construction.

A few years later, at a conference for medical professionals that the CFIDS foundation organized, I discovered how this strange list of symptoms came into being. When we read the list a few months before, we were confounded by the symptoms the agency had chosen to list. Rarer symptoms were listed first, some prominent and common symptoms were left out entirely, and the experience of the illness, its gestalt, its felt quality, was not on the page. Midway through the conference, when the representative from the CDC had finished her presentation, someone from the audience rose to ask her how the agency had come up with the official protocols for diagnosis. She answered the question almost casually. The symptoms, she said, were chosen and listed randomly.

Random choice. The image I get is of wandering symptoms, like characters in search of an author, disparate and shapeless with nothing at the center. The method may make sense if you are doing a survey. You would want to pick names from a telephone directory almost blindly, for instance, if you are studying public opinion and wish your results to be uncontaminated by your own opinions. But in the life of the body symptoms are never experienced randomly. They come in clusters and, grouped together, form a kind of coherence that can be sensed. The cluster of symptoms, for instance, that you feel when you are coming down with a flu. As one sensation is added to another—headache, fever, fatigue—you begin to grasp the nature of your affliction.

Though if you did not know the name for it, you would not be able to diagnose yourself as having the flu. This is where a doctor's knowledge is crucial. In the realm of healing, perception is achieved through collaboration. It is a democratic process of a kind. Even to name the symptoms, doctors and patients must work together. A doctor may ask you to describe what you feel, for instance, but if you have learned no words for the symptoms you are experiencing, you may not even have delineated them. While I was very ill, I found it difficult to read. But though I am dependent on reading for my work, I never listed this difficulty as a symptom. I assumed it occurred simply because I was so fatigued. Even when a friend with the same illness told me of the cloudy spots in her vision, blotting out letters, words, sentences, I did not realize that I had the symptom. But later, after talking with her, the spots appeared again, and finally I could see them. It is a phenomenon I first understood from Wittgenstein, the philosopher of language, who pointed out that a sunset will not even be perceived until the word for it is learned. We need words not only to describe what is observed but to observe at all.

And there is this too, bearing both on medicine and democracy. What you are able to say or even know about your own experience depends in some mysterious manner on the attitude of the listener. Truth comes into being by call and response. The curiosity of the listener is like a magnet, pulling testimony from an inarticulate obscurity. And as with any tale, when the listener has heard the story, the process of telling will be healing in itself.

Deprived of your own authority, you will be tempted to look toward another authority to tell you what to think. The same process that occurs between parents and a child or governments and citizens also occurs in a doctor's office. Whether the attitude of your doctor is abusive or simply paternalistic, if you are not seen and heard, your faith in yourself will be shaken. Somewhere in the breach between your own knowledge and medicine's ability to apprehend it, you cease to trust the knowledge of the body. As you pass your authority to others, whether it is a doctor, a nurse, a laboratory, or hospital, you are hardly aware of the loss.

And this too is a collaborative effort. You may be very willing to forfeit your authority. Illness is wearying. To have someone else take charge, someone who knows more than you, can be a relief. If you have been sick for a long time or searching unsuccessfully for a cure, you will want to believe a doctor who says he can cure you. Even if you grow worse under his care, you will tend to deny what your own experience tells you. After Marie Duplessis's death, Liszt told this tale. He referred her to a doctor popular among society women, but under this man's care she grew worse rather than better. Yet she did not question his procedures until she grew gravely ill. It was only then she discovered that, using an experimental treatment, he had been slowly poisoning her with strychnine.

Faced with pain or the fear of death, everyone tends to look for omniscience if not omnipotence from their doctors. And the reverse is also true. The ability to heal others is associated with divine powers. I am thinking of Charles X, the king Alphonsine observed as he retreated through Normandy. He was crowned in the year that she was born. Following tradition, he chose the ancient cathedral at Reims as the site. Then, like so many kings of France who came before him, once the crown touched his head, to seal the legitimacy of his reign, he reached out his hands to touch the heads of his subjects who suffered from scrofula and who believed they could be cured by a royal touch.

To place yourself in someone else's hands can be soothing. It would be like surrendering to a lover. To trust is part of the pleasure. You can feel the healing in your flesh; it is like being blessed. Still, not every lover can be trusted. The transgression may be subtle. The way a lover looks at you, for instance. Not meeting your eyes, perhaps, or sizing up your body as if it were an object. Then you find yourself growing unresponsive, as if your body knows that to yield would be to betray yourself.

Fundamentally, medicine has a diminishing view of the body. There is an unspoken pornography at the root of the philosophy that diminishes flesh: the idea, inherited from science, that matter, including the human body, is of its nature spiritless. A thing. Perhaps the container of the soul, but only that. You can feel the tincture of the thinking when you are a patient. It is perhaps why so many of us are afraid of hospitals. Like certain ideas that the rich have about the poor—that the poor are less intelligent, for instance, or less sensitive—this philosophy leaves the way open for cruelty.

By the same tradition, not just the body but bodily knowledge too belongs to a lower order. Not only is the patient's testimony by definition subjective and therefore scientifically inferior to the seemingly more objective opinions of professionals, but sensual evidence itself is deemed by science to be untrustworthy. Francis Bacon, father of the discipline, puts it more bluntly; ordinary experience, he writes, is "a loose faggot, and mere groping in the dark." Once head of the Star Chamber that tried witches, he must have been aware of the pun. Faggot. The term was used then to refer both to homosexual men and the kindling used to burn them for the sin of sodomy. You can almost feel the breath of an unnamed fear and loathing in his language. And what was the fear? I suspect it was simply all that the body knows.

Chapter 3

When Tiredness Gives Way
to Tiredness

Joan Nestle

Since 1978 I have had a body that marks me as medically queer—in May of that year I came home from my teaching day, kissed my lover who was busy opening Lesbian Herstory Archives mail in the living room, and went into our bedroom to change my clothes. I bent to remove my black pumps, felt a little dizzy, and collapsed. I remember a terrible coldness and my voice saying, "Deb, you better call the doctor," and then I came to on the floor of our bedroom.

For the next ten years I visited doctors in an endless search for what was devastating me, for what was causing the night sweats, the dizziness, the heart arrhythmias, the mental confusion, the sore throats, the headaches, the muscle pains, but most of all, the fatigue that would swallow me up. I remember doing a very simple thing, shopping in a supermarket with my lover, and suddenly, the blanket of tiredness smothered me. I hung over the shopping cart, knowing that without its support I would have slid to the shiny floor. How strange it is that as a way to summarize the years of illness, my mind throws up this image of a sudden assault in the midst of an everyday task, but that was the burden of this illness, to keep doing all the things that constitute normal life while I was drowning. For ten years, I struggled to keep my life afloat, doing all the things I had to, all the things I wanted to do in the world so I could feel that I was more than a chronically tired complainer. I taught, I wrote, I demonstrated for gay rights, I made love. And I visited doctors.

I had decided early on in my visits to doctors that I would tell them I was a lesbian. This illness was the most personal thing that had happened to my body since my first experience of lovemaking. How could I ask them for help to unlock what was clearly a medical puzzle and not tell them of my life? I was not naive about the medical profession's long history of homophobia; I had come out in the late 1950s when the pathology model of homosexuality was considered the height of scientific thinking about same-sex desires. My mother had reported back to me her doctor's response to her fears that I was a lesbian. "Don't say that," the doctor had said. "That's like saying your daughter has cancer." The year was 1957. But in the 1970s, when we were fighting so hard to change the way the professions understood their gay clients, I thought things would be different. What I did not understand was the limits of the medically frustrated mind. Over and over I was told, "You are depressed. How is your home life?" I was already deep in the shame of this unexplained illness that was driving me to ask for more medical attention than I ever felt entitled to in the first place and now added to the mix was the old shame again, the illness of being queer. One doctor, a highly recommended Park Avenue hotshot, young and liberal, asked me to write a short biography and bring it to his office for our first meeting. As usual Deb came with me. She sat in one high-backed leather chair and I in another as the doc put his boot-clad feet up on his desk and read my words. The opening sentence I had written was, "I share my life with a woman." In a short while, he put the page down, stepped out from behind his desk, and approached me. "I know what you need," he said, and bent down, took my face in his hands and kissed me on the lips.

We left his office numb with our rage, unfortunately silenced by our own intimidation and sense of futility. Anyone with CFIDS knows this journey of endless doctor visits, endless medical suspicions of one's sanity, an endless return to a wracked body that has failed once again to make itself understood. The fact that I did it as a lesbian only marked my exile from the known world with a heavier hand. In 1981, after an extensive blood test, I was told that my Epstein-Barr titer count was very high and, given that I had had a bad case of mononucleosis as a college student, I fit into some unclear possible category that was under medical construction at the time. This illness had scarred everything it touched—my relationships, my job, even my writing style. Too tired to concentrate for extended periods of time, I packed all I wanted to say into short intense pieces. As the years passed, I learned to live with this chronic state of "feeling poisoned," as one woman had so powerfully put it at a Long Island support group. I saw doctors as problems came up, like high blood pressure or headaches, skin rashes or stomach pains, telling them when they took a history that I had chronic fatigue syndrome or whatever name it was being called that year. Some just laughed and said there was no such thing; others said, *we have no idea what that means.* I settled into a pattern with my managed care doctors, some-times giving them copies of the books I had written, jokingly prom-ising not to thank them in those public pages. My gayness, like my strange complaints, became part of a benign relationship.

I had learned that all I could do as a patient was report what I was feeling and then hope my doctor would take me seriously. Some-times we would both laugh at my overflowing medical chart. I was always anxious about not being too demanding, not being too queer as a patient or as a woman. Unfortunately, all of this was to be my undoing. In 1996, I started to have severe stomach pains—or so it felt—and other digestive problems. I started to feel sicker than I had ever before. Standing in front of one doctor whom I used as my last resort because he was familiar with CFIDS, I questioned him if his diagnosis of my stomach pain, "stomach upset," could explain the severity of my discomfort—and he, giving me one of those "here you go again" looks, said *yes.* I asked him if he thought I needed a colonoscopy, but my records showed I had had one the year before. No reason for another. And he would have been right if the doctor who had done the colorectal examination that year had not rushed the exam so. Two months later I was severely anemic and a week after that blood was pouring out of me. I had advanced colon cancer; no longer confined to the wall of my transverse colon, the tumor had eaten its way through the wall of the colon into the fatty layer of tissue that is the last line of defense for the abdominal cavity.

The surgeon removed half of my colon; the oncologist gave me a year of chemo. The doctor who had missed the tumor wept at my hospital bed. When I was feeling strong enough I went to see him in his office. "I don't know if it was because I was a woman or a lesbian, but at some time you stopped listening to me," I said. "I don't think it was because of those things," he said, "but it was because of this," and he held up my thick medical folder that had been given him by my internist. "You had too many complaints," he said. In a catch-22 moment, he said later in the conversation, "You should have complained louder; the squeaky wheel gets the attention." Then I saw the figure of CFIDS standing in the office with us. All the years of both trying to be a good girl and not annoy the doctors too much and all the years of trying to take care of myself in the face of unexplained symptoms had led me here.

Even during my year of chemo treatment, I tried to make sense of things. I asked the oncologist if anyone had done research on the effects of chemo on patients with CFIDS. The answer was a flat *no.* I felt like I was raising the question of a ghost. Now I had a real disease, a killer disease. Why did I want to bring this problem child into that world with me, why risk my credibility as a cancer patient by reminding doctors that for so long I had been a medical suspect? I think now, should I have gone to a gay doctor who would not have thrown my lesbianism into the problem pot, should I never have told doctors I had CFIDS? Which secret would have made me a more respectable patient?

I had been schooled in my acceptance of a failing body by my over twenty years' experience with CFIDS. I learned to slink away from doctors and return to my controlled life in my own community, rationing out the good hours. Now I have two exhaustions vying with each other for my kindness of response. I do not know anymore where the CFIDS tiredness ends and the cancer exhaustion begins. I do not know anymore where the CFIDS patient, so used to so little, ends and the cancer patient begins. I do know that I was set up for inattentive medical care by my long years of shame about being the complaining lesbian woman. Tiredness is a complex thing; it starts in the cells and ends in the spirit. It becomes a reflection of all our failures. *Fight,* I am told, *fight the cancer.* But I need to rest first.

> *Postscript:* After reading this over, I want to add that while I was not taken as seriously as I would have liked by the doctors of the past, I still had better medical care than 99 percent of the people in this world. And my present doctors are trying as hard as they can.

Chapter 4

Object Assembly

Floyd Skloot

The most pronounced deficits were overall IQ; visual sequencing; nonverbal problem-solving ability; visual, spatial and fine motor functioning.

Dr. Sheila Bastien
*Neuropsychological Deficits
in Chronic Fatigue Syndrome*

They were five fingers and naked
fist palm down. They were wooden
bones too long in the grave, middle
and index still joined, the rest
adrift. They were a puzzle simple
as stark truth. He scattered them
before me, an offering from my own
future I could not assemble in time.

Nor could I assemble the Africa
that was a face without sense
organs, perhaps ears and nose
islands to the southeast, eye
afloat near Cape Verde. Time
was up before I found Madagascar.

Then I remembered summer dusks
spent shifting shades of blue
and red, hours finding patterns
centered around faded lilac
that became fields of fleur-de-lis
as jigsaw shape fitted to shape
and the familiar picture grew whole.
Monet came together in half
the time the box allowed.
My son, now the age I was then,
slapped hands across the card
table. Those days time was never
tight and my brain was intact.

Half a life later time reminds me
the temporal lobe scarred by virus
no longer functions as it should.
Rooms have walls in surprising
places and I get lost where I know
the way. These are called deficits.
Tests that would be games some other
time focus on what I cannot do.

So a Doctor of Psychology packs
the disassembled objects away beside
his blindfold and blocks I failed
to place in slots on a formboard
fast enough. He turns back to me,
knees to knees, flipping pictures
that have something missing I am
to name. I think the door should
have a wall around it but learn
later it should have had a knob.

Perhaps it is his face void
of expression, or his cracked
black bag of toys, or my young son

floating again near me with one
cerulean corner of sky cupped
in his palm. Perhaps I am tired.
But these tests at last reduce me
to tears like a child schneidered
by his father at gin rummy.

PART II:
ATLANTIS

Chapter 5

One Window

Dorian Key

What I really need to talk about are the windows. They have become an obsession with me, not my windows, but everyone else's because I have only one, a narrow but tall window looking through a darkish corridor between our building and the one next door. So, my need for windows has grown slowly like a canker, emerging under my tongue quietly, forlornly, and small, until like a stone it anchors heavily my entire bottom jaw, which is open and drooling for more glass, more view, more light, more life. For my life is often a quiet solitary one, one of little activity and much staring and gazing out of my one window. I look out this narrow view of life I have until I feel I am suffocating within the narrow echo of the long walls of the buildings that frame my view. I drag myself from my bed and with shaking hands I assemble an odd outfit of whatever lies close on the floor and haphazardly garbed I beckon my always-companion, my service dog Monroe, who steadies my pace by letting me rest my hand on his back. We go down the street, past the usual herd of drug dealers and buyers, past the wandering homeless and the scrappy pigeons, past the scatterings of trash to the muddy, soggy park. While I lean up against the chain link fence surrounding the soccer field with my hands stuffed in the pockets of my well-mended jacket, my dog runs about sniffing and wagging his tail, as glad as me to be out in the cold fresh air. I look up at the sky, so much bigger here without the buildings to hem it in, but then it is the buildings my eyes are really drawn to. Buildings with bay windows, rows of tall narrow windows, and small ovals of glass peeking out of attic rooms. Victorians and Edwardians mostly surround this neglected park in my part of the city and I yearn for my own building with lots of windows, with unlimited views, for life to look out at and a building to feel secure in, but not trapped by.

When Monroe has finished snuffling about and returns to my side and when my nose and cheeks are stinging with the cold air, I decide to head back. When I finally settle back into my warm bed, clad again in flannel pajamas with a cup of tea to sip, I am able to rest contentedly in my large room with its disproportionately small window. I am able to enjoy the warm constraints of my comfortably furnished room, even though it has only one, and a small one at that, view of the outside world, for now it is enough. Although today I was lucky and I managed to make it outside, often my life is much narrower, as I am trapped inside my flat day after day.

Having one window is a lot like having a disability. My view, my outlook is limited by a chronic illness, by physical constraints, by narrow parameters. Forced to rest, to remain in bed, to cancel plans time and time again, unable to hold down a job, staying in bed a lot of the time, I cannot help but get restless. I am forced to find ways to escape, to travel in my head, to dream while awake and while asleep, to live as fully as I can in a body that cannot go very far. Since I can't experience the outside world firsthand very often, I cannot touch and revel in it, rolling and romping with it like my dog playing in the park; I wish to have more windows to open. I wish to see the world from more than just one angle, to sniff at it and read its temperament, its personality, its movement and feel, like my dog does when he climbs up on my bed, licks my face, and then pokes his nose through my room's one window. For a long time I was covetous of my roommate's front-facing bedroom with its four windows, and I avoided going in her room, for it would remind me of what I did not have, just like being around too many healthy people with their expansive lives and their secure pretty homes. It made me think too much about what I had lost, the life opportunities, by being ill. As long as I stayed away from the reminders, I was usually okay. But still for a long time I dreamed of knocking a hole in my one outside-facing wall that cried out for an opening. Tara and I talked costs and building codes, of convincing the landlord that we could put in a new window, but in the end when our building went on the market we decided to wait on making any more investments of our time and money. So I began moving forward by not taking outward action. Because time and again I am forced to practice movement while staying still.

My friend Helene and I used to say to each other that being sick wasn't as hard for us because we liked to lie around and read, to watch TV, to have large amounts of time to ourselves. I had other friends who weren't as lucky, who couldn't stand the slow, almost immobile pace of watching rain come and go, of listening to cars pass and the murmur of people, laying back in an almost trancelike space zoned out with a fever or exhaustion, occasionally waking to read or watch a bit of TV, or perhaps talk with a friend on the phone. And then there are those days when I do get out, and am able to do quite a bit, when my energy is pretty good. Oh what wonderful days those are. When I am with someone like my friend Christopher, also ill, we thrill at the sights and sounds of our city like country folks, visiting for the first time. "Look at the cars!" I exclaim. "So many of them, and the people!" We lean back in our chairs at an outside café and laugh and comment with delight. As it is to just-released prisoners, the world is amazing and beautiful to us, even in its most mundane details. Sometimes when I am by myself I find myself smiling and nodding at the drug dealers in front of my house, my heart almost bursting with the joy of seeing another human being in my long days of solitude. Occasionally, we chat about the weather or my dog. I find myself using my limited Spanish to speak with the old Latina sweeping the sidewalk in front of her house. Maybe they think I'm a little nuts, but they are always polite and smile back at me, indulging me like a small, neglected, starved-for-attention child.

My mother once said to me, "It's like you suffer from arrested development" and she's right. I've spent over twelve years being sick, often feeling older than I really am, but not always really, fully growing up. Being forced to live in my narrow, one-view world, often confined to bed, like an elderly invalid, I have grown old before my time. But unlike most elderly folks, I don't have a vibrant, productive young adulthood that colored and molded my days to remember fondly. Still, when I have days of some energy my youthful self takes over, my arrested stage of development little kid runs wild and escapes through that one window, my door to the world, breathing freely and carelessly loving every minute and every breath and tremor in my body.

Chapter 6

Silent Trespass

Nadine Goranson

I woke up on a Thursday in early May, and couldn't get out of bed. In fact, I couldn't move. My muscles ached and my throat burned. My sweat-soaked body shook with chills. The kids were about to start their summer vacations from school, work was busier than usual, and I had a long list of projects ready to accomplish during the warmer weather. It wasn't flu season, but it sure seemed I had a doozy of a bug.

I called in sick and settled myself on the couch with a good book and the remote control. Two days off, some more rest on the weekend, and I'd be back in business. But by Monday morning I still wasn't feeling right. I had trouble breathing and walking up the stairs and to the car. Waves of heat poured over my body, leaving me dizzy and weak. I decided that getting back in the swing of things might be good for me; surely this was just the last of that pesky flu. Tackling pantyhose and getting two kids off to school, I told myself not to overdo things this first day. I didn't. But by 2 p.m., I was back in my car, pale and hot, driving home to fall into bed.

Within months, I would count myself among the disabled.

Leaves fell, the temperature dropped, the snow melted away. Still, I did not return to work. In fact, I went from five years of full-time employment to "taking a couple of weeks off" to placement on leave of absence to, finally, termination—all within a three-month span. Full-time job with benefits, mutated into disability and noninsurability—just like that. My doctor began by treating me for an upper respiratory infection. We ruled out mononucleosis, thyroid problems, and Lyme disease. We looked for "bugs" I'd never even heard of, like cytomegalovirus. We even looked for cancer. After a barrage of blood samples, X rays, urine specimens, ultrasounds, and more, my doctor gave me some confusing news.

"I believe you're developing chronic fatigue syndrome," she said.

Chronic fatigue syndrome. Okay—so I was really tired—who wasn't? In fact, for the last month, I'd been bothered by extreme insomnia. It was ironic—sleeping in the daytime, then eyes wide open at night. Someone suggested I just had my "days and nights mixed up." I needed a schedule, I needed to get in shape, get more fresh air, but I couldn't get out of bed.

With those thoughts, I began my struggle and search to learn all I could about the debilitating illness that calmly and quietly slipped into my life and changed the rules. It would be a long time before I planned a weekend—or a day, for that matter. Chronic fatigue immune dysfunction syndrome (CFIDS) forced me to live life one day at a time, one moment to the next.

In the United States alone, it is estimated that about 800,000 people are afflicted with CFIDS, though many may be misdiagnosed or not diagnosed at all. The condition brings with it not only persistent, debilitating fatigue, but also recurring mild fever, sore throat, painful and swollen lymph nodes, unexplained generalized muscle weakness, muscle and joint pain, severe or unrelenting headaches, confusion, inability to concentrate, depression, forgetfulness, photosensitivity, and sleep disturbances such as sustained insomnia, night sweats, and chills. Calling this illness "chronic fatigue syndrome" is like calling stomach cancer "chronic stomach pain."

My case was somewhat typical, though no two people with CFIDS have the exact experience. The symptoms came, one by one, sometimes two by two or more. There was no pattern. In the beginning, each day was a mystery unfolding—what would I feel like today? Well-meaning friends offered to take me out to get some fresh air and sunshine. I just wanted to be able to get up and go to the bathroom, or maybe make it up the stairs without running out of breath. CFIDS took charge and threw me into bed for the day, or allowed me to get up, only to experience waves of heat and a screaming sore throat. Going to bed at night was an adventure in restlessness. If I was able to fall asleep, I woke each hour, shaking and soaking wet from head to toe, reeling from vivid high-action dreams—"crazy-making dreams" my support group would later call them. Friends brought me books; I was too exhausted to read. My brain wasn't able to focus. I couldn't see the words, the paragraphs melted together. I felt like I was living underwater.

After awhile, the onset of new symptoms seemed almost ridiculous—impossible for one person to experience so many in a given week. I began to keep things to myself, afraid people would think I was a hypochondriac, or worse, a lazy bum. Time passed, and as I began to be able to get out of bed, I worried that I wasn't really sick at all. Maybe I was crazy, or lazy. As the weeks dragged on, I found that if I put some concealer over the dark circles under my eyes and rested a lot, I was able to go out and accomplish an errand or two on a good day. A trip to the post office or bank became an accomplishment. I decided to make one trip out of the house each day, to force my way back into life, back into the stream. I'd walk slowly through the grocery store, leaning on the cart, or spend some time at the library, looking for any information I could find on chronic fatigue syndrome. But always with my throat sore, my muscles aching, and my determination beaten. Often disoriented, I finally had to give it up and get home to rest. Eventually, I spent most days at home as my symptoms waxed and waned in an unpredictable jumble.

My husband took over on the home front. He drove the kids to school, cooked dinner, took care of laundry, did the grocery shopping. All the tasks we had maneuvered around both of our busy schedules now had to be crammed into one busy schedule, while my daily goal was to get showered and dressed. We discussed what it would take to keep our household going and delegated additional chores to our thirteen-year-old daughter and seven-year-old son, explaining that we all had to pitch in a little more to keep things running. I felt overwhelming guilt. It was bad enough to be unable to work at my job, which had given me an identity, provided wonderful friends and challenges, and rewarded me with a paycheck. Now I couldn't even take care of my home, my children were confused and scared, my husband was run ragged. I felt helpless; my life felt out of control.

After twelve long weeks, my employer was no longer obligated to hold my position open for me, and I received notification that I would be terminated. I jokingly referred to it as the "T" word when talking to friends—secretly, I feared what lay ahead in this newfound life of mine.

My benefit package had included disability pay, so I was okay financially for the time being. However, the medical insurance I had carried for five years with my employer was cancelled upon my termination. In fact, my entire family had coverage under my plan, and their policy was cancelled as well. No more employment; no more insurance. I checked into the COBRA plan guaranteed by law to continue covering employees for eighteen months after termination. I was told it would cost me over 700 dollars each month for the same family coverage through the COBRA plan. It was out of the question.

I searched for help, certain that I was simply uninformed, that I would find affordable, comprehensive medical insurance for my family and myself. After all, I had always been a good employee; I had always paid my share of our insurance premiums through payroll deduction. I was no slouch; I worked hard and paid my bills. But nobody could help me.

First, my husband insured the entire family through his employer's HMO; the premiums were higher than we were used to, but we needed the coverage. We paid, but there was a catch: anything related to my illness would not be covered. Preexisting condition became a new phrase added to my vocabulary.

It didn't make sense. I had paid for medical insurance in case of an illness. Then I became ill and lost my medical insurance with my job. I didn't blame my employer; it was just the way the system worked. Now my illness was a "preexisting condition," preventing me from getting sufficient medical insurance. What kind of system was this? It seemed like a mixed-up circle of impossibilities. I decided I just wasn't informed enough.

I made phone calls, asked questions. Finally, I called on a friend I had met through my job. He was well respected in the community, and had worked in the insurance field for years. I knew he would do all he could to help me—and he did. He referred us to an agent who could offer us an affordable comprehensive policy for the entire family. Our problems seemed solved. Because CFIDS is a chronic illness, the symptoms are long term, but usually require little hospitalization or emergency services. The agent seemed relatively certain there would be no problems getting our medical insurance.

He was wrong. Our application came back approved for my husband and children, but I was rejected. I called several other agencies—

with no luck. Finally, a very compassionate insurance agent told me over the phone that I had an "uninsurable" condition. In short, no one would insure me—because I was sick. I could quit making phone calls.

A final possibility came from a friend at work. She was aware of a state program for uninsurable people. I received information from the Colorado Uninsurable Health Insurance Plan (CUHIP), and, out of desperation, signed myself up. My premiums would cost more than twice the amount we would pay for my husband and children combined. We made too much money to qualify for Medicaid, but not enough to afford this. I took the chance anyway, hoping we could make it work.

I was told I would have to go through a six-month waiting period for all charges stemming from my preexisting condition. In other words, in addition to the high premiums, we would have to pay for prescriptions, doctors' office visits, and any other medical expenses related to my illness for six months. After that, they would consider my charges and pay a percentage of them. I realized a couple of weeks into it that we just didn't have the money to maintain the expensive policy while paying for all of my medical expenses ourselves. A month after I signed up, I called to find out about temporarily canceling my policy. The woman I spoke to told me that if I cancelled, I wouldn't be eligible to apply for coverage again for a year and a half. I gave up. I cancelled the only possibility of health insurance I had. I simply could not afford it. I found it ironic that my entire life I had been healthy, and I always had health insurance—now I was sick, and no one would insure me. For the first time, I understood how a person could "fall through the cracks" of our health care system. I understood that health insurance was for the healthy, and those who could afford it.

Over time, CFIDS symptoms realign themselves in a different fashion for each individual, changing on a daily, weekly, or monthly basis. In my case, after a few months the sore throat diminished, muscle aches became more intermittent, and my energy level improved somewhat. Instead, I found myself dealing with short-term memory losses and confusion. I lost my way to the local library; I forgot entire sentences midstream in conversation. I used the wrong words and drew a complete blank while talking. I forgot what I was talking about, even forgot the names of people I'd known a long time.

My mind betrayed me, so I became my own watchdog. I questioned what I said as I was saying it, repeated names and topics in my mind while trying to listen to others. I became disoriented in department stores and confused in conversations. People I knew well became uncomfortable around me. Like a new kid in school, I felt out of place and unsafe.

I also began gaining weight for no apparent reason. My size ten body slowly put on pounds, regardless of what I ate or didn't eat. I began to feel embarrassed about my appearance, and each time I became a larger size, my self-esteem plummeted. Not only could I not do anything, I didn't even recognize myself in the mirror any more.

Losing contact with friends upset me more than I had expected. Of course, I never imagined the number of people who would simply disappear from my life—people I had spoken with on a daily basis for five years, people whom I had even met with occasionally outside of work. In the beginning, I felt cared for and missed. Co-workers brought casseroles to my home, donated paid time-off hours to help me with my declining income, and called often to see how I was doing. The goal of many of those early days was to write thank-you notes to every single person who remembered me.

But CFIDS is not a convenient illness. In fact, CFIDS affects lives in a way that is particularly contrary to our society. Today, what a person does tends to define who a person is. CFIDS patients are generally not able to *do* much of anything, especially in the early months of the illness. Our business world is goal-oriented: we identify the problem, assess options, and begin taking steps to solve it—then move on to the next. Project management. Accomplishment. Control. CFIDS changes all that and makes people afraid. As a person with CFIDS, I was afraid, wanting to regain control, but unable to do so. People with CFIDS often describe the illness as a roller coaster: terrible days when muscle and joint pain are extreme, memory loss is continual, and even breathing is difficult; good days when a shower and a trip to the store seem a joy, a reason for celebration; the in-between days when the struggle goes on inside, the patient determined to get out of bed and *do* something, even though it hurts. When friends saw the randomness and lack of cause-and-effect logic the course of my life had taken, they too became afraid. Soon, phone calls diminished and encouragement dwindled.

Some rationalized that I had not kept in touch with them. I had more time on my hands than they did—I was home all day. Couldn't I pick up the phone? What they didn't understand was that I couldn't. They didn't understand the debilitating fatigue that caused me to lay in bed for hours, unable to pick up the glass of orange juice on my nightstand next to me. They didn't understand that my brain didn't work the way it used to. They didn't understand that I wasn't simply tired. I tried to explain the fatigue to them as the "anesthesia wave," likening it to that moment right before surgery when you realize you're about to lose consciousness. I thought that might help them understand its severity, and my inability to "fight it off." When I explained the additional symptoms, almost too many to believe, some thought surely this was a mental health problem. Some thought it a convenient excuse to escape the rat race we all complained about over lunch in the past. Some told me I was lucky to get it and be able to be at home, "not really sick, just enough to stay off work." Some told me they wished that they could get something like CFIDS. Eventually, my illness and I simply didn't fit into their busy schedules. My swift recovery date had been pre-dicted and changed—an erasure on the calendar one too many times. My personal roller coaster had taken on a life of its own. The phone calls dwindled and eventually almost stopped completely.

I also fought the battle of my goal-oriented upbringing. What pur-pose could I create for myself to justify my existence if I was unable to *do* anything? What good was I? Like many other thirty-somethings, I had questioned my life's purpose long before the illness struck. At least I had choices then. I realized it would require a drastic change in my thinking patterns to get the answers to these questions now. I worried that I might never find them. I couldn't help but remember the com-mittee meetings at work when we had discussed the need for a "para-digm shift" in order to survive in the changing world.

As strange as it may sound, my paradigm shift came when I quit fighting my illness. About a year into my illness, I remember resting on the living room sofa one afternoon as the sun filtered in through the sheer curtains and hanging plants, splotches of sunlight dancing across the tapestry rug. It was my favorite time of day in that room. As I noticed the warmth of the sun and the shadows it cast, I realized for the first time that I wasn't doing anything. I wasn't worrying about money. I wasn't questioning the meaning of life. I wasn't foggily planning an herbal attack against my latest symptoms. I certainly wasn't moving around. I wasn't sad or happy or frustrated or angry. I just was.

With that realization, I then quickly reminded myself that I had a terrible illness and that I wasn't doing anything about it. No stoic affirmations churned in my head. No mustering-up of energy. No medication review. And I realized, surprisingly, that life went on. Without my fretting, figuring, and fighting, life went on. Life went on, and so did I—but suddenly without the fear, without the anxiety, without the guilt. It was just life—not a contest, not a race, not an accomplishment. It was just my life—and CFIDS was a part of it. I realized the CFIDS and I were going to have to learn to get along together.

That was well over a year ago, and CFIDS is still a part of my life. I'm no longer wearing pantyhose, except on the most special of occasions. I can't work at a job because it would take me three hours to get ready to go (and then I'd probably get lost on the way there). I still have what I call "days from hell," but I also think I've learned to notice a little bit of heaven right here on earth. I can hear the birds now, singing on a spring morning, and I notice grass growing up through the cracks in the cement. My plants get watered now and misted. I so enjoy the way they respond to care as opposed to the neglect and frustration they got from a hurried and frazzled working mom. I appreciate being able to pick up my glass of orange juice. I relish being able to read again, even if only for a few weeks at a time. A call or visit from a friend is such a treat—I notice them now, the nuances in their speech, the laugh lines around their eyes. Of course, in between are days of pain, disorientation, and fatigue. But each day is new; each moment is unique. I live each moment as it comes, and realize that I never really had control anyway. I no longer cram my desk calendar with lists of urgent tasks. I take life one day at a time.

In fact, I think that tomorrow, I'll wake up.

Chapter 7

Prisoner of CFIDS

Mayra Lazara

UNO

When I was a tot I flew with my aunt and brother from Cuba, the pearl of the Antilles, to Miami, fleeing Communism. My parents had departed first and were anxiously awaiting our arrival. Back then, I thought Communism was some sort of poisonous chemical that would seep through my brain and cause permanent neuron decay. I heard that America, the place we were headed, produced slutty blonde women who dared to smoke cigarettes and would constantly engage in sexual encounters, while the men were all amoral sexual perverts and drug abusers. Imagine the fears I had before landing in this ever-so-perverted territory.

Our family had been aghast when they heard that Americans threw out their clothes after wearing them only once or twice. We were astounded. So, my understanding back then had been that being around "immoral, degenerate, and wasteful" Americans was far better than the possibility of my brain going into spontaneous combustion from Communism. Fleeing one prison to live in another was not my idea of having fun. Little did I know what kind of prison truly awaited me.

DOS

I saw my world in America as a beginning pastel watercolor that easily changed tones by a mere stroke of the brush. My inexperience and innocence had me in a continuous state of exhilaration, wanting to closely inspect, survey, and ask questions about everything. I had that constant itch to learn new things. Life was an unpredictable exaggeration of claylike megastructures waiting to be remolded, by me, with insurmountable energy.

I lived in constant acceleration, always a step ahead of my Cuban neighbors, as if I was made of pure electromagnetic energy. I was never a sickly child, but rather an overactive one. If I felt ill, I wouldn't mention it to my family and would secretly go out to play. I always fished for tadpoles, watched my neighbor pluck her live chickens, played with my best friend, Changi, climbed trees, rode bicycles, skated, played baseball, did the hula hoop, jumped rope, slid on the slip-'n-slide, and had a million other diversions. I had sufficient energy to light up all of Miami. Even when I, and all my neighborhood friends, caught the chicken pox, I managed to run out and play. Illness would never bring me down. As I grew into a teenager, my excitement and exhilaration for life became even grander.

TRES

In my twenties, desire to become independent and leave my Republican xenophobic culture was of utmost importance. I gravitated more and more toward leaving my home, family, and culture, to take a voyage into the unknown. My mother, whose values were massively different from mine, thought my leaving home was crazy. The implications were that I no longer loved my family and had a gravitational attraction to an American lifestyle that would certainly keep us apart forever. Maybe, they thought, I had to move away because I was a Communist! They couldn't understand my energy and zest to live my life to its fullest.

I had to fill my void and off I went, with my energy well packed, continuing upward, constantly trying to learn about homophobia, xenophobia, capitalism, vegetarianism, Buddhism, Marxism, environmentalism, and a few more *isms*. I predicted great things for myself and for the world. I started my voyage in Boston with infinite energy and enthusiasm. I was ready to uncover and discover, ready to live to my fullest, to meet friends, travel, find love, and to live out all of my dreams.

In Boston I worked as a hairstylist while going to school, and played the djembe (a handmade Senegalese drum) in a women's African drumming band. On some weekends, when I wasn't creating hairstyles, I'd hike Mt. Monadnock, in New Hampshire, with friends. There were times when I drove on my own to Miami, around 1,500 miles, to visit my family for a weekend, then drove back with even more energy and exuberance to get back to hiking the White Mountains. After a few years of working, going to school, having loads of fun while walking, jogging, driving, hiking, and enjoying life, I collapsed. I figured I had overdone it. *Too much walking. Too much hiking. Way too much driving back and forth from Miami to Boston,* I'd tell myself. *With a little rest I'll be back on my feet in no time,* or so I thought.

I've never gotten better, no matter how hard I've tried. I've been ill seven years. I used to have only four symptoms: dizziness, fatigue, severe exhaustion, and migraines. Now I'm up to twenty-five. I've run out of fuel. A million times I've tried to resurrect, to no avail.

CUATRO

Let me tell you what it's like to be me now. In the mornings, when I awaken, I can't stand up because my blood pressure drops and I faint. I'm up by 7:00 a.m. but need to stay in bed until 11:00, with a bursting bladder, due to the fact that I can't get up to use the bathroom. Mornings are the worst.

I've set up a small refrigerator next to my bed. As soon as I open my eyes, I grab a piece of bread and small carton of soy milk. This way I won't get a hypoglycemia attack. I eat while lying in bed. I then force myself to take my mind off my pain, exhaustion, nausea, and inability to stand up by reading the paper or meditating. Once I've tried to sit, I need to stay in that position a while. If I abruptly get out of bed without having been sitting, I will undoubtedly drop from the vertigo and orthostatic intolerance. When I feel I'm ready, I can then try to stand while leaning firmly against the walls. The bathroom is just five steps away, but it feels as if I have to painstakingly cross the Great Wall of China to get there.

Sitting on the toilet is an ordeal because my thighs and knees hurt from fibromyalgia. Sometimes when urinating, I feel faint and must force myself to finish quickly. I hurriedly brush my teeth while urinating. Luckily, the toilet is next to the wash basin. At that point, standing up is excruciatingly difficult. I hold onto the walls again. If the room is spinning, I try not to vomit and shuffle back to bed as carefully as possible.

Once I've rested for about three hours (walking to the bathroom and urinating takes it all out of me), I'll get my laptop, place it on my stomach, and read my e-mail. I then try to write a letter to my pen pals. Sometimes, after writing them, I'm so exhausted I begin to shake, shiver, sweat, and feel brutally cold, as if I were standing nude in the center of the North Pole. I'll grab my sweatpants from under my pillow, and reach for my sweaters and leather jacket on my nightstand. Once I'm all bundled up, I must lie there, like a mummy, completely covered by a burning hot electric quilt, until I thaw out.

It's normally a balmy 90 to 100 degrees out in the summer. I lie there wishing I could walk outdoors and melt like cool ice under the scorching sun. Usually my thawing takes about an hour, but afterward I'm left sicker, weaker, and in much more physical pain. When I'm done baking, I become so hot I'll rip off all my clothes, throw the blankets on the floor, and lie naked in bed with the air conditioner at fifty-five degrees and a fan soothing my body, absorbing my sweat. Heat and humidity intolerance are two of my most painful symptoms. I feel as if I'm on fire.

Paradoxically, the more I rest the more tired I am. So after lunch I always try to walk to the recliner in the living room. I become increasingly exhausted and out of breath. My peripheral neuropathy becomes heightened, and sometimes I can't walk at all due to its severity. When I *can* walk, I'll hold on to furniture to rest, then continue moving. I must. For a moment I'll stop and, if possible, try to stretch. One stretch and I feel I'm going to collapse from exhaustion and severe burning pain in my arms. By this time, nausea, depletion, throbbing neck pains, and inability to breathe sets in. I have to try to walk to the bedroom as soon as possible or I'll black out from pain and fatigue, as has so often happened. Sometimes I make it to the chair and recline for half an hour.

This has been my routine every single morning of my life for the past two years. Before that, I could walk half an hour or do yoga, as long as I rested a great deal throughout the day. I could go shopping for small items. I could even shower every single day, as long as I napped. It's obvious that my CFIDS has gotten worse.

CINCO

I've tried everything imaginable, from meditation and visualization to megavitamins, deep breathing, healers, reiki, massage, relaxation tapes, Western and Eastern doctors, Santeria, sanctified waters from La Virgen de Guadalupe (something my mother brings from her travels), medication, supplements, rest, exercise, etc. Exercise means brushing my hair with one hand first, then the other, while sitting on the bed.

What I *can* do is enjoy visual stimuli. The immense window in my room overlooks my lush backyard. I marvel at the pregnant banana trees, the mangoes, papayas, limes, guanabanas, oranges, grapefruits, and figs. I feast my eyes on all that I can absorb. I usually have a gut-wrenching urge to zoom outdoors, film the iguanas, pick bananas off the tree, climb coconut palms, and sway from their fronds, then lie naked under extreme Florida thundershowers . . . but I can't.

I now have vertigo every day. I can shower once a month if I'm able to sit on the shower stool, but it must be fast. Bathing is extremely difficult. My body usually aches so much that soaping myself hurts. I can't use any hot water whatsoever, due to the severe heat intolerance. For me to shower, I must stay in bed all that day and not even try to sit up. There have been times when I haven't bathed in three months, mostly during the winters, because the water is too cold and my body can't handle it. I can't even use one drop of hot water or the fainting spells and extreme heat intolerance will worsen.

Be assured that if I'm not severely ill, I try my best to bathe. Every single day I want to bathe, but can't. So I'll lie in bed imagining a magical rug taking me far into the vast jungles of the Amazon where I visualize bathing in cool spring waterfalls.

I can no longer pick fruits off my trees. I easily pass out from trying to walk; it brings on extreme fatigue and peripheral neuropathy. I must continue my struggle to feel better.

SEIS

I have flashes of swimming in the crystal-clear ocean, like I used to, of jogging and bicycling twenty miles over the Rickenbacker Causeway to the sea (as I did most Saturdays when I first arrived in Miami), and of working. I long to continue my landscaping design job. I crave, with body and soul, to design, then dig in the dirt and install huge swaying palms, all sorts of trees, plants, and flowers.

I feel a great need to be able to walk again in order to rediscover life, but I get paler, weaker, fainter and fainter until the vivid canvas of what my life was gradually becomes erased. *We're in the year 2000!* I keep telling myself. *We're technologically advanced. They'll find a cure.* I'll be able to walk, run, climb, drive, eat all kinds of foods, exercise, talk for over five minutes without feeling as if a Mack truck hit me. I'll be able to travel, play with my dogs, shower standing up, go to the movies, play my guitar, eat ice cream, go hiking, and swim in the ocean. I'll be able to hug people who are wearing perfume (I have severe chemical sensitivities). I'll be able to horseback ride, work, dance, play drums, sit up and watch TV, water the plants, kayak, and do all those things that make me feel human.

SIETE

CFIDS has maliciously taken everything from me, like a thief stealing from the poor and deathly ill. My memory no longer functions properly. I have to rest while brushing my teeth because my arm muscles hurt so badly. Brushing my hair exhausts me. Petting my dogs for over a few minutes leaves me completely drained. I can't pick up a dish to eat from because it's too heavy (I eat from paper plates), and the fibromyalgia will kill me a few hours later. I can't even shear a tiny shrub because not only can I not stand for long periods of time, but the excruciating pain in my muscles won't allow it. Sometimes, due to swollen, painful, axillary lymph glands (under arms), I'll get high fevers and can't move my arms.

I used to feel like a star, shining bright, but I now feel as if I am getting dimmer and dimmer.

The constant pain in my spleen is a reminder that I can only eat one mouthful every three hours. My migraines are excruciating. My bones, muscles, and joints constantly hurt. Sometimes I ache so much I think I'm dying. My body is wasting away because I can't exercise or digest food well enough. Doctors have thought that I had lupus, multiple sclerosis, heart failure, a brain tumor, lymphoma, and leukemia. My CFIDS resembles all these illnesses and more. I'm in the percentage of CFIDS patients who get sicker and sicker.

OCHO

I want to sit out in the sun with my family and friends and talk, eat handpicked sun-splashed fruits, and hose down *mis amigas* with liquid laughter. Talking for brief periods of time brings forth extreme exhaustion, so I haven't seen any of my friends in about two years. I haven't seen my brother in eight months. He thinks I don't love him, but the effort and hardship of talking and having company exacerbates all my twenty-five symptoms. I don't want my family to suffer, so I try to keep them from seeing me deteriorating.

I'm one of the lucky ones who has the most giving and loving life partner in the history of the world. Perhaps I'd be dead if it wasn't for my partner, who massages my frail aching body, who continuously tells me that I'm going to heal, who meditates and prays for me, who helps me with anything I need, and who allows me to be independent because I can't imagine it any other way. (I must get up and walk to the bathroom on my own even if I know it might kill me. I ask for help rarely, such as when I have all twenty-five symptoms at once, and can't even sit to drink a sip of water.)

I've wept many times, and grieved for my health, but always find things to keep my mind off my illness. I make up anagrams, do crossword puzzles, read humorous books and joke books, read the paper, pet my dogs, watch an hour of entertaining TV a day, meditate, stare out the window, and write. I can't allow this monster to rip me apart, so I will continue to do what my health allows me. *I want to live! I want my life back!*

NUEVE

I don't have insurance (they don't accept anyone with preexisting conditions). I was denied by the Social Security Administration twice because I couldn't get to their doctor due to not being physically able to walk past the door. Sitting is more of a problem, so a wheelchair would make no difference at all. I'm so frail I can easily pass out after sitting for over a minute. The way I could make it to their doctor would be on a stretcher, but it would be too costly and stressful to call an ambulance. Last month when I phoned my doctor he said, "You need to be hospitalized. I am at sea with you and your illness. Call Dr. Nancy Klimas. She has a bag of tricks for CFIDS." I felt as if he'd shot me in the stomach then threw me in a garbage bin before kicking it to the curb. I need a doctor who's an advocate to help me get an environmental illness-safe ambulance and hospital room, not someone who discards me.

I've begged, supplicated, and pleaded for the SSA to please send their doctor to me because I'm bedbound. To no avail. I've supplied them with numerous letters from my personal doctors and sent them my blood results, which state clearly that I am disabled by CFIDS. To them I just have delusions. *How on earth can anyone be so sick and not be dead? She must be lying! Chronic fatigue immune disorder syndrome is a hoax!* I can hear them thinking. Honestly, though, SSI must think that CFIDS is not a real illness. Otherwise, how could they not have helped me after knowing how ill I am?

DIEZ

I get by even if I have no job or income. My mother brings me food on a daily basis, helps me monetarily, and supports me by believing that this is a real illness. She's seventy-three, goes out dancing on weekends with her husband of eighty-three, travels the world, and runs errands. Every time I see her and her robust health, I'm reminded that I'm the old decrepit one.

Who would have guessed that what I had to fear in America, while flying to my freedom, high over the tropical Cuban rain forests, was an incurable illness? I've been expelled from my *home*—my body—by CFIDS, for a prolonged period of time. I've been captured, held exiled by the enemy who continuously keeps me in pain. I'm confined and deprived of pleasures, and of the quality of life that should be everyone's birthright. CFIDS just won't let me go. I am a prisoner of CFIDS, but I will fight to release myself from its shackles, even if doing so kills me!

Chapter 8

Bittersweet Nightshade

Floyd Skloot

It has been months since I could walk this far.
At noon the fencerow thick with bittersweet
nightshade flashes with summer sun. There are
no clouds, no fleeing deer, no swirls of breeze,
nothing I remember from the last time
I was here. Now I lean my cane against
a post, lying back where the long stems climb
and scramble over everything that rests

in their way. I love to see these blue stars.
Their five points bend back to reveal a blunt
golden cone nestled in the heart of leaf
where in this light long shadows run like tears.
The wide yellow berries starting to run
toward red are the exact color of grief.

Chapter 9

Right Where I Am

Kate Foran

I walk around my neighborhood in the morning, and it is beautiful. The sky is a blue that goes on forever, the air around me is alive, and the sun filters gently through the unfolding leaves. As I turn a corner, something catches my eye from the short spikes of grass pushing through the dirt. It is a glimpse of blue, a robin's egg, like a piece of fallen sky. I haven't seen one in a long time. It's been so long since I've been *able* to walk and find a robin's egg, and I realize I've been aching to see just that shade of blue. I pick up the delicate shell and rest it in my palm.

I am thankful for walks on spring days as I recover from this long illness. I dreamed about such things as I lay on the couch, hardly able to make my way around the house.

I first became sick with chronic fatigue immune dysfunction syndrome just before my fifteenth birthday. I was so young, a child really. I was unscarred by any real hardships, unprepared for the pain, fear, and confusion I would have to face. Like a weak and tiny bird that had to struggle to break through its egg, I had to struggle through this illness.

It was a struggle in every way. It was a struggle daily to survive the head, joint, and muscle pain, the dizziness, the complete and utter fatigue. It was a fight to somehow keep a mind clouded by memory loss and brain fog active and engaged. It was a battle to accept this new definition of myself as *sick*, and to face the fear that I might never get

---

"Right Where I Am" by Kate Foran originally appeared in *Youth Allied by CFIDS*, Fall, 1997, published by the CFIDS Association of America. Reprinted with permission.

better. It was a struggle to preserve my spirit as the world as I'd known it—all my plans and dreams, my very sense of myself—fell apart.

"This is not the way," I often uttered, especially in that lonely hospital room with the too-cheerful pictures on its grayish blue walls, the metal beds, and view of the parking lot. I wanted to be anywhere but in the midst of sickness, blood tests, CT scans, SPECT scans, and cardiograms. I wasn't supposed to be sick. I was supposed to be normal, like everyone else, complaining about school, sitting around with my friends, laughing.

I was sick for most of my high school years. I couldn't go to school at all, until now, what would have been my senior year. I am not graduating. I have accepted this fact, so that it does not prick me anymore when I hold it. But it is a fact; I will not wear a cap and gown, will not march with the classmates I have known for thirteen years, will not receive a diploma. It seems as if my high school years barely began, and now they're over. Now I must shut a door I hardly opened. There is no ceremony to help me do it.

So I think about what I've lost and what I've gained. Sometimes it is hard to know where this experience fits in with my life, and where my life fits in with this experience. It is hard to know where my experience fits in with everyone else's.

I think of all of this as I walk with the eggshell held out before me. I pass an older couple and a young woman. They are standing in their driveway next to a car with luggage piled inside. They all look sad, especially the couple. The young woman hugs first the man and then the woman. They are saying good-bye.

I feel awkward walking through the scene, like I don't belong. But then I look down to see the broken eggshell in my hands. I smile as I realize the connection. The young woman is leaving the nest and I am marching through with a broken egg. I am a part of this; I belong in this impromptu ceremony, even though they're not aware of it.

It is then that I realize this can be my ceremony, too. I have broken through to a new beginning. I have graduated; this is the way. I keep walking, with that bit of sky resting in the nest of my palm. I belong here, right where I am.

Chapter 10

Valley of Shadows: Journal Entries

Phyllis Griffiths

Saturday

At least twice today the entire world faded to gray for a few moments. It does not blur so much as fog up. The fog comes and goes with the level of fatigue. It may be a seizure manifestation. I do not wish to lose my sight. I don't think I could cope with that.

Friday

The fatigue continues to grow. I am exhausted. The psoriasis on my arms is angry and sore. My skin feels grainy, as if covered in sand. Nerves jangle, and muscles twitch and jerk. A spasm, a twist, pain, weakness, dizziness, collapse. Unable to move, unable to not move. I want to be held and cuddled. The people around me ignore me, avoid me, wish me to leave them alone. Too weak to make supper, I am resented. I resent the resentment. I resent the abandonment. I resent the thanklessness of my life.

Saturday

Sounds of traffic drift into the room. Motors growl, tires moan and squeal. The neighbor's shop yields up sounds of work—a bang, a clunk, the rapid "brraappp" of an air wrench. In the other room the fish tank bubbles. Someone sharpens a blade—the sound of stone on steel. The night is hot. Too hot to be bearable with the doors and windows closed to block out the sounds from without. The silence will come soon enough. I need but have patience for it. The motor sounds echo far in the still air, sounds from speedway race cars. The roar reminds me of the howl of the wind that chills my soul with fear. I am uneasy with this sound. I wish out to cry out for quiet—but cannot.

My body longs for restful sleep, easy sleep. The stress I feel is crushing, smothering, oppressive as heat. I close the bedroom door—and the sounds of the family fade. Time grinds by as I sit. The closed door dampens the breeze and the heat builds. It builds like the stresses build. One at a time—one added to the others. All demands. No concessions. Hoops to jump through and loopholes to fall through.

Sunday

Depression haunts me. I feel sad and weak, unable to do much of anything at all. Part of me truly wants to get busy and clean up, bake, do laundry. But even trying is beyond me. Weakness prevails, and in its wake are guilt and sorrow—and shame. Of course I feel depressed. Each time I try to do what I once did, I fail. My body fails me with weakness and pain. My mind fails me as I lose focus and memory. Circumstances bring crisis after crisis that take all my energies and abilities to cope, leaving me drained for days to come. Motivation leaves, anguish comes.

Thursday

I sit here not knowing what tomorrow will bring. Money is a real problem. Lack of money is a sore point that festers all the other problems like flies around an open wound. My body gets weaker and my symptoms increase. I am afraid that I will never get stronger now. I want to hope, but I have little left but acceptance. I must face my greatest fears. I dread what must come next, if all is to come into play. Aloneness, suffering, being uncared for. Abandonment on top of help-lessness. Oh, how I fear that fate.

Saturday

I am afraid to admit to the family just how weak I am, that there will be no change in their attitudes, and that would hurt very much. They already neglect me and deny me aid. I fear that soon I won't have any choice in this regard. My body does not respond to my will. Today I can barely walk at all.

Tuesday

The pressure in my chest grows and I feel like lashing out in blind fury at my plight. I don't know what to do. Once the rent is paid and Don's work expenses are put aside there will be nothing left but empty cupboards.

Friday

I feel like I am in a black hole. It seems I can't draw energy from anywhere or anything. Like I am really not here at all. I have more strength in my dreams than when awake. There is no reserve, no reprieve. Nothing at all of anything. Less than empty. How can that be? Yet that is the sensation I feel. Hollow, fading, collapsing into itself. To curl up and disappear. Too weak to fight and too weak to care. Only fear in the form of panic breaks the silence, flames that cry out—unheard—for help. I can't even tell Don what I need. I can't think of what I need. My mind is as weak as my body.

Thursday

Don's unemployment benefits are finished and I don't know how on earth or in hell I can cope with the ever-increasing hardships. I pray to God for help. Welfare is the answer? Argh! But I can't get well on welfare. I'm scared witless. I can only function by focusing in on the now. Otherwise I'll break and I will surely die.

Friday

I am deeply depressed, even suicidal. I hate being filled with so much fear and worry and dread. I feel sick all the time. I am not even strong in my fantasies anymore.

Wednesday

I told Don off tonight. He dismisses my suffering as less than his own while he is far more mobile, stronger, and energetic. I push myself to my limits every day trying to do as much as I can to take care of the household and myself. He doesn't make himself ill for days doing anything on my behalf, but he doesn't think twice about dragging me about when I'm too ill to feed *him* when he can't make use of the meager resources in the cupboards. And then to be faced with Don's disdain, disgust, avoidance, and neglect—not to mention denial and minimizing—if I complain or even try to gain recognition of how ill I am.

Saturday

I was quite ready to die tonight and maybe I still am. I was ready to go wild and trash the place. A little push and it would have occurred. I am tired of staying alive simply not to inconvenience others. I am weary of it all, especially the uncaring, self-centered arrogance that I have to put up with from my husband and sons. I'm crumbling fast. I feel like a slave. I am a prisoner of my illness and a slave to their needs.

Sunday

They do not seem to realize how humiliating it is for me to have to beg for help; how humiliating it is for me to be unable to do things. They shame me for asking, for being dependent on them. No matter how much I cry or explain they still punish me with their scorn. I feel like an unworthy piece of shit, asking them to inconvenience themselves for me. As long as I do not inconvenience them, they may consider cleaning up their own messes. I feel very dirty in my being, an unwanted burden upon their lives.

I longed for the peaceful release of death this night. Lois (another young adult we have taken into our home for awhile because she needed shelter) just came in my room demanding to know what's bugging me. I asked her to leave and she wouldn't. I yelled at her to please go away and leave me alone. She got hostile. This is the only place I have to hide and I want to be left alone. I had to yell at her to leave me alone. She finally left when I grew hysterical. I wish I could lock the door. I really wish I could. I wish I could find a place that was safe and warm and comforting. I just want not to hurt.

I went hungry again today. I cried for it. I couldn't get up the energy to cook up a potato or a pot of rice or oatmeal. Those were my choices, but I couldn't see the instructions and I was too ashamed to ask for help. All I get is improperly prepared foods, which make me feel worse, and glares of resentment. When I did attempt to go for supper, to have some chili, I fell over Don's work boots in the hall. They were hidden in a shadow and I banged my toe so hard even my hip hurt. I had asked to have "dangers" removed from the floor earlier in the day, and when I attempted to do so myself I was shoved away under protests of "Let me do that." Then I had difficulty seeing, and I managed to avoid Mike's boots only to slam my foot into Don's.

After the cramping in my foot and leg stopped I again tried to make it to eating. Everyone was seated and out of the way so I wouldn't fall over them. As soon as I reached for the back of Don's chair for balance he pulled it in. Again my left side was jolted as I banged my toe on the chair leg as I stumbled. I got to the counter for support and burst into tears. I could barely make it to my room to cry. After calming down I made my way back down to the kitchen. Don offered to make me something but I refused. I can produce burned toast and cold tea with no problems and no resentful looks either.

Later, I cried at Don and Mike. I told them that I am humiliated by telling people over and over again what I need and what is wrong. The same foolish questions are asked and answered endlessly and nothing ever changes for long. I tossed Don my binder of ME material and I told him I have an equally large one on fibromyalgia. Damn it all, I wish he would read and understand. I am so tired of pleading for consideration. It is humiliating to have to beg all of the time. To exist at the convenience of others.

And I am expected to just put up with this quietly.

And so I did not die, not all of me anyhow. The body that held my spirit did not die even though the spirit of the person I knew as me no longer lived. I was deep in mourning for the self I had lost, and it seemed to me that nothing was left but the empty shell that now chained me to a painful existence.

Chapter 11

Stealth

Willy Wilkinson

I was born at four minutes to midnight one balmy September night in the Year of the Tiger. Close to the edge. When my mother was pregnant, my Popo* looked at her belly and knew that I was a boy. Everyone said I was going to be a boy. At her baby shower my mother pulled a long black hair off her head and strung her wedding ring on it to see which way it pointed, and that, too, indicated that I was going to be a boy. But just as I was the surprise child arriving years after my other siblings, I took them by surprise that day. I wasn't the black-haired boy she was expecting, but an auburn-haired girl. My mother named me after a Chinese actress she admired, whose name translated into a common 1960s girl name. I hated it.

I am *hapa*. Hapa comes from the Hawaiian expression *hapa haole,* meaning half white. My mother is Chinese from a tiny little nowhere town in Hawaii; my father is English, Irish, and Scottish from Oakland, California. I am pinks and browns, freckles and burnt skin. I am Chinese eyes with epicanthic fold, flat-nosed, small in body. I am boy in girl, man in woman, compassion, intuition, language, rebellion, swagger, butchness. I was born on the edge of race and gender.

Though in many ways my mother was a strong community leader, she made a point of shuffling her feet for her great white husband. Yet my feet were firmly planted in the soils of my choosing. When I was four years old I decided that I wanted to be white and male. I figured that was the only way I could have any power in the world, so I decided that was what I was going to be. I created a fantasy world

---

*Cantonese for Grandmother.

where I imagined myself white. I imagined myself a boy. I thought if I tried hard enough, I could become that, and the world would perceive me that way.

At nine, I changed my name. I passed as a boy sometimes and I loved it. "Are you a boy or a girl?" was the playground refrain. I embarrassed my parents; I freaked people out. When it comes to gender, people just really need to know what you are. And they get so flustered when they think they goofed. But as far as I'm concerned, the joke's always on them. Today, well into my thirties, I still pass for that boy and I love it.

I didn't realize I was a woman until I was eighteen. Though I had hated women all my life, I began to realize that I loved women. It was a difficult time. I was never going to be the good Chinese girl that my mother so desperately hoped for. But coming out into a largely white lesbian community, I struggled with being tokenized, disregarded, and ridiculed. When I was twenty I began the process of coming into my identity as a woman of color. I began organizing Asian lesbians and lesbians of color on the West Coast, East Coast, and in between. I networked locally, nationally, and internationally. I wrote articles and edited a newsletter on Asian/Pacific lesbian issues. The time was ripe. Many of us were isolated, and as a community we were struggling for support, empowerment, and visibility.

In my mid-twenties I started working in public health. I conducted street-based AIDS education to high-risk populations on the streets of San Francisco's Tenderloin, Chinatown, and South of Market Districts. Drug addicts, sex workers, homeless, whoever was out there. I loved it. There was something about sitting down with regular folks and stopping the spin enough to say, hey, your life is your business, but whatever you do, be safe. I pioneered an AIDS prevention outreach model that specifically addressed the needs of the Asian and Pacific Islander community. It was the 1980s, and there was a lot of work to be done.

Though I have been a leader in many communities, as a mixed heritage person I have not always been welcome. My "realness" has been called into question. All my life people have drawn attention to my ambiguous looks. My cultural experience has been disregarded. Strangers have stopped me on the street to tell me that I dyed my hair. People have been sure that I was one thing or the other, or something else altogether. They have told me who I am and been disbelieving of who I've said I am. At times I experience generic racism; other times white people have tried to "white bond" with me, to get me to participate in their racism. Or they've tried to use me to assuage their white guilt.

The thing about mixed people is that, like transgendered people, we are stealth. You don't always see us coming, and you can't be so sure about what you're dealing with.

When you're mixed, you're basically on your own. I have found home with many different peoples and I have also felt essentially homeless. I see it from all sides and I get it from all sides. I am accustomed to cultural conflict and surprise with the same intimacy that I know the terrain of my features and the hues of my skin.

So in some way, when I got sick at the age of twenty-nine, I was not surprised by this new dichotomy. There I was with a debilitating illness that was not supposed to really be happening, looking good when I felt horrible, a woman of color with a "white girl disease."

To be sure, I was devastated. I was one pissed-off jock; I mean, my bicycle was part of my body. I was as able-bodied as any of us come, and I couldn't get out of bed. My life stopped, my community disappeared, and once again, I was homeless. Homeless in my own body. Sure, I had a place to crash. But the landlord couldn't fix a thing. It was like lying in some old car whose engine could hardly turn over. Doctors told me I was crazy, and my friends were nowhere to be seen. I lay hauntingly alone while the world passed me by. That was the summer I died.

And yet, how fitting to become disabled with an illness rife with ambiguity and complexity, one whose very realness is questioned. It's the story of my life.

Years into this global epidemic, we are still treated as the pariahs that people with AIDS once were. Like other perplexing illnesses, CFIDS is steeped in controversy and pervasive disrespect. While countless researchers have clarified its essential nature as one of immune dysfunction rather than the result of depression or any other mental or emotional imbalance, CFIDS struggles to be recognized and addressed by the powers that be. Medical doctors and government entities alike dismiss the severity of this illness, particularly because it is so difficult to pinpoint. Fears about possible contagion fuel our outlaw status. There is no one entity that has been isolated as responsible for its cause, nor is there a magic bullet that will make it all go away. How do we quantify the "debilitating fatigue" that relegates so many millions of ambitious people, mostly women, to our beds? And while we may look good, thank you very much, this illness sure ain't pretty.

But you see, people with CFIDS are also stealth. We might look like the average Joe, but we're here to remind others that not everyone can work insane hours and go sailing on the weekends. Like cats, we have a sixth sense: we smell things that others may not be aware of. We signal the toxics in our everyday lives—the foods, the pollutants, the chemicals that make us sick. Our awareness heightened, we are sometimes the sharpest tools in the shed. Other times we drift in mental fog, our words as jumbled as incoherent dreams. We are technological advance gone awry, a twentieth-century conflict raging in our bodies.

I watch and learn from my cat. She sleeps even more than I do, and she couldn't care less. Cats are real role models for these hectic times. Besides, busyness is so overrated.

Over the years my health has improved with a balance of rest, detoxification, and the pursuit of my goals. In my case, I found that I had mercury and other heavy metal toxicity from botched dental work. I have spent thousands removing toxic dental amalgams from my mouth and working to detoxify my body, and slowly, my symptoms are improving. I know a lot of us try every stumpwater from the cemetery–vitamin–supplement–pill–cure–New Age Louise Hay philosophy we can get our hands on. And there are certainly plenty of people ready to prey on our desperation. Some of that stuff can help. But more than pouring all that into the vessels of our bodies, I think recovery is also about emptying the vessel. Detoxification is one of the keys to recovery from CFIDS. And not just on a physical level. I'm talking about removing the toxic people and thoughts from our lives. Free your mind and your ass just might follow.

When I first fell ill, I struggled to do the spiritual work that I needed to do in order to see things differently. Being sick has taught me to weed out the undesirables in my life, to kick out people and things that waste my time and energy, to get the gist of things, and to let go and move on because life is too short. Moreover, having CFIDS has meant that I can't hide from any part of myself. Two years into my illness, I came out as transgender. It meant coming to an understanding of my gender identity as inextricably linked to my mixed heritage. Ultimately, that meant not choosing sexual reassignment, because I am not one gender or the other. Over time I synthesized my complex gender identity and realized that I didn't have to be the gender that anyone else expected me to be. Being sick like that—staring at death on the ceiling—has its way of forcing one's honesty.

Then, sure enough, who should come around the corner but my true love—sweet, smart, sassy, and outrageously silly, a woman who accepts me for everything I am. On the day we got married all the static I've ever experienced was rendered ridiculous and fell away. Enveloped with love and support from our families and friends, I stood ever so proudly on top of the mountain. All the ambiguity and complexity of my life focused itself clearly in the singularity and sureness of love.

In the meantime, stealth bombing continues. People with CFIDS know the war zone really well. We mapped it. We learn how to make tools out of what we've got, and to live with what we're missing. We make the best of those sweet precious moments when all seems right again. And we hope for the future. All I know is, I have found many a shiny stone in this gray, cold place. I have tasted spirit nectar that I never would have known had my world not been shaken so. But the bitter was like nothing I ever could have imagined. It left a nasty, pungent aftertaste. The journey is long and far before we can lay to rest our status as pariahs in this invisible battle.

Long ago, when I was young and able-bodied, I rode my bicycle across the United States. My biking partner hated the hills, but I loved those long methodical climbs. With each revolution of the pedals I pushed my body and soul just a little more. My biking buddy would stop along the way and say, "I just want to *be* there already." That's how I feel every day about living with CFIDS. But somehow along the way I have come to realize that recovery is not just the being there, it's the getting there. And somehow, somewhere, I can accept that.

Chapter 12

Roller Coasters

Eva Marie Everson

I remember that, as a child, I loved roller coasters. I had no fear inside me. The larger they were, the more frequently I rode them. I always jockeyed for the front seat. I loved the anticipation as I slid in and felt the iron bar secure me into place. I grinned as the train jerked forward; laughed out loud as it tipped backward, making its way up the first hill. I looked up at the blue sky and white, billowing clouds . . . waiting . . . waiting . . . waiting . . . until, on command, the train stopped. The riders behind me screamed, but I squealed in delight and raised my hands high over my head. Then suddenly, *vrooom!* Down we went, up and over, tight curve to the left, tight curve to the right, then slowly up another hill. By this time I was nearly doubled over with laughter. I never wanted it to end.

I remember the night, as a young woman and charge nurse in the nursery of a large hospital, I said to one of my nurse's aides, "I don't feel well." The lymph nodes in my throat were swollen. I had a low-grade fever and a mild headache.

"You should go home," she advised. "Get some sleep. You'll feel better by tomorrow night."

But I didn't. Two days later I was in an isolation room with an ominous diagnosis: *rule out spinal meningitis.* They did, but it took me months to recover. This was my third spring in the hospital. Two years earlier I was hospitalized with a severe case of mono; the following year with a severe case of the flu. Now this . . . this what? Final diagnosis: *viral infection of unknown origin.*

I remember the day, twelve years later, when I sat curled on the sofa with my palms wrapped around my coffee mug as I watched the

Oprah Winfrey Show. The guests were the victims of "the yuppie flu," an unidentifiable illness whose chief symptom was fatigue. I laughed. "Yeah, well I'm tired, too," I scoffed. "Get a life."

I remember May 1992. I worked full time, ran an orderly home, had an active daughter and a husband who was wonderful in every respect but one: he rarely helped around the house. It was not unusual for me to be mopping floors at 5:30 in the morning or folding warm, fluffy towels at midnight. I also kept a very busy social calendar, but, just like those roller coasters from my youth, I thrived on the 100-miles-an-hour, twenty-five-hour days I kept. Naturally, when my mother-in-law became ill that month and was hospitalized, I took full charge of her care.

"Nana" was placed in a new wing of the hospital. The strong smells of paint and carpet hit me like a wall upon entering, but it only took a few minutes to get past it. She was released eleven days later, and on the twelfth day I plopped onto the sofa in our family room and declared to my husband, "I don't feel well."

"You're just tired from all that's been going on," he said.

But something inside me said that it was more than that.

By the first of June my life was upside down. I hardly slept. I was exhausted, but sleep evaded me. Everything I ate made me violently ill. I was becoming confused and disoriented. I had splitting head-aches and muscle discomfort. Because I had stuck myself with a few dirty needles during my career in nursing, I began to worry about HIV. One morning, as I tried unsuccessfully to make my bed, I slumped to the floor, pulled the phone off the bedside table, and dialed my doctor's office.

"I think I need a physical," I told the receptionist. She informed me that the first available appointment was December 31. More than six months away. Too tired to raise a complaint, I took it.

But a week later, I called again. I had lost over twenty pounds in seventeen days. My house was a mess. I hadn't cooked anything more difficult than Hamburger Helper in a week. I was beyond exhausted, and still I could not get enough sleep.

"Why didn't you say so?" the receptionist asked.

"I dunno," I whispered. "Just get me in."

I remember the rest of the year as though it were yesterday. I was in a lab, a doctor's office, or a hospital outpatient center nearly every day from July until the middle of November. I became more ill with every passing day. Though my blood tests showed that something was wrong, they didn't say just what that something was.

I remember the night I lay on my bed and weakly turned tear-filled eyes to my husband who lay beside me. "I'm going to die," I said, "and they aren't going to know what is wrong with me."

I remember how helpless he looked.

I remember the day when my doctor smiled at me and said, "We have a diagnosis." Then we talked about the Epstein-Barr virus and my medical history, including the three years of mono-flu-whatever and the new paint and carpet that could have triggered the virus.

That was six years ago. I remember every detail of every up and down. I remember days spent in bed, hospital trips, tests, tests, tests. I remember verbal abuse from doctors and nurses. One doctor was more concerned that I wasn't working than with the fact that I had been battling an ear infection for eight months. I remember the anguish of hearing friends tell me they didn't "believe" in chronic fatigue syndrome. I remember an insurance company that stopped covering me. I remember the days when I woke feeling better . . . actually feeling better . . . and doing too much . . . and the next day being worse.

I remember roller coasters, and laughing out loud, and sneering at Oprah's guests, and walking four miles a day, and not being able to walk across the room, and working from sunup to sunup, and a brain made of cotton candy and blood made of dishwater, and the sweet smells of summertime and the pungency of new paint and carpet.

I remember all of this. But I don't remember feeling well.

PART III:
MEMORY AND METAPHOR

Chapter 13

Immune Means Memory

Kathleen Bogan

1.
My mother hurls herself to her knees
on the spotless kitchen floor, arms raised
in a kind of praise, or to get
my attention. It works. Sure
she has me transfixed,
she clasps her hands, wails "Please, God,
don't let me hurt her."

2.
The doctor speaks slowly, with certainty,
with a kind of clinical reverence. His voice
comes to me through a fog: The purpose
of the immune system
is to remember, to recognize an invader,
even one in disguise.
To marshal armies of lymphocytes, activate
antibodies, to kill off the threat.
With no sense of metaphor, he composes
an etymology: Immune means memory.

"Immune Means Memory" by Kathleen Bogan originally appeared in *Writers' Forum,* Volume 21 (1995). Reprinted with permission.

3.

"Immune" is derived from the Latin *immunis,* meaning not common, but exempt. "Memory" has a different etymological root altogether: *memor,* or remembering. The word following "immune" in the dictionary is "immure," to shut in with walls, seclude, or confine. The next word is "immutable," unchanging.

4.

The kitchen drawers
are my mother's arsenal,
stocked with tools that slice, shred,
peel, grate, squeeze. I am forty
before I know
why these drawers,
in any house,
make me uneasy.

5.

Children in this country are losing the ability to think in the abstract, the counselor says. She works in theater now. She tells children stories. Told the tale about the lion and the mouse, about how the mouse saved the lion by pulling a thorn from its paw, children used to grasp happily that the story means little people can do big things. She says this. Now, she says, about the lion and the mouse children are very concrete: the lion is scary, the jungle is scary, things can hurt you. She says this is not what the story is about.

6.

No one believes our stories,
till we're older. Black eyes,
broken bones, the shadows of violence
in the depths of children's eyes, no one sees
till we're older.
Till we know the right words.
Or our bodies talk.

7.
You know how the immune system works
when it goes haywire? It no longer differentiates
between self and non-self, between what is foreign
and harmful and what is related
and familiar. T cells and B cells mistake body
for enemy. We fight ourselves
when no one else does.
We devour our strength.

8.
First there were aches, fevers,
lumps that felt like my armpits had been torn open
and softballs sewn inside.
Arms, legs, neck, knees, feet, inflamed,
were poor receptors for feeble messages
from my brain. I scrambled left
and right; nerve synapses, like hands
reaching across space, missed, plummeted
into the void. Words eluded me, or floated unsupported
in the hazy sky of consciousness, refusing to be tied together
into sentences. In the concrete world I could barely function.
Asked to explain the importance of a free press
in a democracy, my mouth and tongue froze.
The doctor made another mark on the scoresheet.

9.
The radio played "Daddy's Little Girl."
Mother sang it, endlessly. I thought she sang for me.

10.
My heart becomes a radio,
relaying signals, wild and fast.
The doctors huddle round my bed;
I'm wired for sound and pictures.
They can't make sense
of what they receive. They let me go
after two days, impressed

but definitionless. They finally decide:
an "irritable spot" in my heart
it sends out its own spark,
in conflict with the spark-in-charge
from the vagus nerve. They don't know why.

11.
What I learned in the kitchen
watching my mother pray: I learned
my mother did wrong things
in the kitchen. I learned she was afraid
of losing control. I learned control
could slip at any time. It was dangerous.
It took prayer to keep things safe. I learned
she couldn't stop. I learned God wouldn't.
I got hit anyway.

12.
The doctor
has a new theory now,
and, boy, is he excited. Epidemiology
is detective work, he says. I think
it's like a game: Colonel Mustard
in the library with the candlestick.
It's toxin overload, the doctor says,
the cumulation of a lifetime
of unhealthy places, unhealthy living,
unhealthy reflexes, and, oh, here's the important
part: they think it's hereditary, they think, they
think it's gender-related, they think the clue
is in the women, they think. They think
the secret answer is my mother. They think my mother
is the instrument. My mother,
in the kitchen,
with the knives.

Chapter 14

The Paradox of Lost Fingerprints: Metaphor and the Shaming of Chronic Fatigue Syndrome

Peggy Munson

In a dusty attic box, my mom has stored a book that chronicles every detail of my birth. Amid newspaper clippings, between facts about the weather and historical happenings, there is an ink print of my palms and the soles of my feet. On the yellowed reports of my birth, the historians breathe a collective sigh of relief when they use the modifier *healthy* to describe me. I know my parents wished those prints of my hands and feet would fix my well-being in time, keep me young and undamaged forever. *A healthy baby girl, her fingertips ten hops of a skipping stone, her palms ridged with long life lines, her feet engraved with the topographical swirls that would mark her distinction.* More than anything, they hoped the sterile hospital room from which I was emerging would protect those personal imprints of mine forever.

But the illness that took over my life at age twenty-three caused one overlooked symptom in a subset of its patients—a perfect metaphor for what it was. Due to a freakish autoimmune-like effect that caused swelling in the hands, it actually *erased* some patients' fingerprints and rendered the skin smooth.[1] Chronic fatigue immune dysfunction syndrome (CFIDS) sanded down the whorls of identity. It made us perfect thieves and perfect victims. Perfect to ignore, easy to blame. Digit by digit, person by person, the erasure deindividuated the very hands that symbolized our humanity, our vote in freedom. But the fingerprints hold a paradox. The smooth fingertips—they seem to tell so much.

They seem to indicate, like blood tests that reveal no dramatic abnormalities or a bird that clutches to his perch until he drops over dead, that nothing is there. But what they tell best is what they cannot tell. They remind us of what has been taken away. In a system of disability that puts the burden of proof on patients, who must compile mounds of evidence to prove to government and society that they are really ill, the smooth fingertips also represent the paradox of CFIDS, an illness that seems—like a criminal suspect—to erase its own evidence.

On the surface, medicine seems to overflow with metaphors. Autoimmune effects, as in lupus—the wolf in red velvet—are an easy parable for the girl who was too greedy, and thus was eaten. Certainly, as I have lain in bed and longed for the woods, I have imagined myself to be that girl. I have—like her—repeated the mantra of date rape victims—"How could I have walked into this of my own volition? How could I have been so stupid?" I wonder if I shouldn't have worked so hard in school, created bad karma, lived exuberantly in the years before I got sick. As the lead in *The Shawshank Redemption* says—after being wrongly imprisoned for years—some of us just walk into bad luck. But denial surges against this notion. I am not a pure fatalist. I believe in my own agency. And I tried to undo the bodily harm. I stood in line at the ambrosia clinic for the misunderstood, swallowing exotic tinctures with names in the kind of staccato translations you see on foreign T-shirts. On feverish nights, the insect of my id thrashed around on its flypaper, disbelieving that it could be so stuck, that I could be so sick. For years, I fought a battle I can barely describe, one of raw and childlike instinct. Keith Jarrett, the jazz pianist who caught this disease, once played a dirge for himself as he felt his body succumbing, sensing he was playing his last concert for awhile. I know this very dirge. It has lodged in my brain with its terrible cycles of mourning. I know when the illness is going to put me in bed for weeks. Playing a dirge for oneself might seem premeditative, but it isn't. It is merely instinct.

CFIDS behaves like an autoimmune disease and also like an immunodeficiency condition. Thus people view us both as perfect victims and as perfect perpetrators. They tell us we have fought too much, subjected ourselves to stress, imperialistically destroyed our bodies piece by piece. They tell us we not have fought enough. We are weak, prone to overstatement, lacking in resilience. After years of contradictions, we too have been cancelled out. We are an epidemic made up of stereotypes, lacking the indelible, assured identity of the healthy. People don't accept the smudge of what we are. They want words. They want lines. And thus, where the ink of our bodies does not delineate, the ink of society draws a caricature that becomes us.

I had no idea that my place in epidemiological and cultural history would play a giant role in the way my illness was perceived. I simply collided with a pathogen. In 1992, on a day in May, the sky started spinning. It did almost seem like something out of Revelation. I fell to the earth, profoundly disoriented, clutching the grass as if it were the hair of a lover. Nobody saw me—not that time, or most of the subsequent times in weeks to come. My witnesses were a few toilet rims and some people who offered to help me get home. Before the vertigo started, though, there were ominous signs. In my apartment, carpenter ants crawled into the center of the kitchen and died, in droves, like the rats in *The Plague* who prophesied the coming tragedy. Certainly, in my own life, I can notice such symbolism. For a year I had been having a hard time swallowing, as a painful lump grew in my throat. I wanted, as much as everyone else, to see this symptom as symbolic and not neurological—something about hindered expression. In 1992, though, when the strange flu struck, the one that was not really influenza but had no better name, I moved out of the symbolic and into the hurricane of my own destruction. In the storm that would become my life, empiricism was truly the eye—a strange calm that had nothing to do with the force of nature. I was no longer an observer of any kind, but a person trying desperately to survive with a shred of my belongings.

In this tragedy, all the people around me seemed to have an urban bystander syndrome. They noticed me and yet continued on with a lilt in their steps. I didn't feel victimized, exactly—I just wanted them to care. They would later read about me, somewhere, in the best papers in the world. They would let the journalists write. For the moment, though, they walked toward their distant towers of production with blithe disinterest. They thought about me on a coffee break, but forgot my true likeness. Perhaps they inserted their tired faces where my face might have been. But this gesture wouldn't be empathy; it would be fear. And it wouldn't be likeness; it would be telescopic nearness, a kind of remote voyeurism. They would read the best newspapers in the world, papers that would create a good story for what they had witnessed. Stories full of metaphor. Stories of biblical proportions and biblical clichés. And then they would make a lesson out of me.

THE HYSTERIANS

Propped up at my computer one day with unwashed hair and devilishly pale skin, I read a book review in *JAMA: The Journal of the American Medical Association* that called my illness one of "the vogue diagnoses of this decade."[2] True, CFIDS had caused me to lose almost thirty pounds, adopt a Gothic pallor and blackened hair, and reversed circadian rhythms that—to the young Marilyn Manson crowd—perhaps gave me a superficial hipness. But many years ago, when a doctor finished up her diagnostic repertoire with a tandem gait test in which I struggled against balance problems to walk a straight line (she called my performance on this test "poor"), I did not feel much like a runway model. Still, a group of academics decided to approach my disability as if it were a trendy craze. The most notorious was Princeton feminist literary critic Elaine Showalter, a bargain-hunter by her own admission, who decided to spruce up her intellectual wardrobe by embracing what Dr. Victor Stenger calls the "fashionable" belief of postmodernism "that all statements, whether in science or literature, are simply narrative."[3]

In an era of self-identification, Elaine Showalter picked up her trademark gold lamé briefcase, walked into a classroom, and declared herself a medical humanitarian. Like a traveling quack from another century, Showalter based her scholarship on a blend of metaphor and myth. She asserted that many conditions, including CFIDS, arise out of a cultural need to belong, to express the inexpressible, and thus people manifest so-called diseases they read about on television, in the newspapers, and in popular magazines. Showalter's voice was like a sudden epidemic, squawking through the talk show circuit to promote her "expert" treatise on the subject of my illness, a book titled *Hystories: Hysterical Epidemics and Modern Media*. Articles quickly appeared about her in *Harper's, Mirabella, The Village Voice,* and *The New York Times Book Review*. Her publisher scheduled her on a ten-city book tour, plus appearances on *Good Morning America Sunday,* Washington DC's *Fox Morning News,* and *Rolanda*. Though one doctor called her book "beyond mean-spirited,"[4] the book jacket reviews praised *Hystories* as "smashing" and "muscular." Strange adjectives, but oddly appropriate, as Showalter became one of a peculiar group of 1990s antiwoman feminists—a kind of wife-beater in drag.

Stating that CFIDS is an outbreak of *fin de siècle* (end of the century) panic, Showalter—educated by the same pop culture venues she claimed caused my symptoms—treated my illness as a social metaphor. She contended that people with CFIDS, along with those reporting alien abduction and various tabloid ailments, had fallen prey to a stream of media narratives, subconsciously absorbing these stories (or "hystories") and using them to explain unusual physical symptoms. *The New York Times Book Review* noted that Showalter ignored the long historical precedent of legitimate illnesses once considered psychological before a pathogen was found. Tuberculosis was once widely considered to be the result of a "tubercular personality," the writer explained, going on to describe a woman in therapy who complained for twelve years of muscle degeneration that left her unable to lift a toothbrush. Her psychiatrist diagnosed it as "repressed rage" at her parents, when she was really developing myasthenia gravis, a disease of progressive muscular deterioration.[5]

Showalter portrayed these new hysterics as people resisting psychological interpretations of disease, desperate to place "cause and cure outside the self."[6] With no concrete research into the physical mechanism of CFIDS, she deemed herself an expert, stating, "hysteria tells a story, and specialists in understanding and interpreting stories know ways to read it."[7] Describing hysteria as "a body language for people who otherwise might not be able to speak or even admit what they feel,"[8] Showalter's tone sounded eerily like that of a racist anthropologist in Africa interpreting tribal dance. With an implicitly bigoted assumption that this subordinate order needed to be helped by academics or psychotherapists, she seemed to see her hysterics—including people with CFIDS—as some kind of tribe resisting progress.

Showalter aligned herself with a class of scholars she dubbed the New Hysterians, some of whom see hysteria as "a sort of rudimentary feminism, and feminism a kind of articulate hysteria."[9] Her book followed the precedent set by other Freudian revisionists such as Edward Shorter, who wrote the book *From Paralysis to Fatigue: A History of Psychosomatic Illness in the Modern Era* (Free Press,

1993). In the late 1990s, as it became popular to criticize political correctness, it was shrewd of Showalter to pretend to be a postfeminist revolutionary. Her new hysteria, however, was not retro chic but recycled oppression, a biased rant against an already battered population. Feminism has often found value in reclaiming derogatory labels and transforming them into powerful expressions of liberation. Showalter even went so far as to agree with a scholar who called the New Hysterians products of the "gender revolution."[10] But her argument lost ground when she turned it against an illness population she knew nothing about, then used literary theory to practice medicine.

But few outside of the CFIDS community gave Showalter scathing critiques, and many agreed with her. Showalter cited studies by Simon Wessely, a psychiatrist who later wrote a book to arm physicians against hysterical patients who might present with imagined symptoms of chronic fatigue syndrome. A *JAMA* reviewer called Wessely's *Chronic Fatigue and Its Syndromes* "ammunition to help end an unnecessary epidemic."[11] Co-authored by two other psychological professionals and published in 1998 by Oxford University Press— years after CFIDS was categorized as a debilitating physical illness in England as well as America—the book treated CFIDS as conceptual and therefore open to debate. Wessely and his co-authors, in taking on CFIDS and fibromyalgia, came "to the inevitable conclusion that, but in rare instances, science and medicine cannot substantiate that either exists as a disease or even as a separate entity."[11] These conclusions were mainly based on the fact that CFIDS patients sometimes present with psychological complaints—like patients of other illnesses such as Lyme disease, syphilis, and viral encephalitis. However, only in the case of CFIDS have these symptoms been selected out from all the others as "proof" that CFIDS is a psychiatric phenomenon.

Besides Wessely's crackpot science, Showalter's book was surprisingly lacking in medical testimony, but she had no qualms about making diagnoses with her doctorate in English. As Dr. Anthony Kamaroff stated, "It is rather like my writing a book about the influence of the Reformation on the work of William Shakespeare."[12] And Dr. Jay Goldstein took the absurd logic one step further, joking that his next book would be titled *The Diurnal Variation of Oxytocin Pulses in Feminist Writers; Neuropeptide Secretion, Signal-to-Noise Ratio and Circadian Rhythms in Literary Criticism.*[12]

Naive to what an impact her work could have on practical medical applications for a suffering population, Showalter still gave a pat First Amendment argument and simply stated, "The worst case is that I'm wrong."[13]

Though it may sound odd for an English professor to talk about medicine, Showalter's discipline had already begun to take a decidedly biological turn. Feminist literary criticism—for years prior to her argument—focused on how physiological differences between women and men affect styles of narrative. French feminist literary scholars created the concept of *écriture féminine*, a style of literature mimicking the rhythms of the female body. Postcolonial feminist theorists focused on the parallels between the colonizing of countries and the control of women's sexuality and reproductive freedom. These explorations became an avant-garde and complex analysis of the way language is a true creation of the physical body.

At some point, though, as theory trickled down into practical applications, a schism developed between the language of the sick and the language of the well. Society went beyond *écriture féminine*, or "writing the body," and in fact began to treat bodies themselves as textual genres, books to be interpreted by half-perceptive laymen. Truly, the body does inspire many stories, and they help us to explain the perplexing physical experiences that we all have. When one considers the fact that genetics may determine intricate personality traits, the narrative of most bodies is perhaps more deeply encoded than current science can comprehend. But these stories still remain part of the body's mysteries. Healthy bodies are an easy story. They wake up, they cleanse themselves, they mend their wounds, and they sleep. Ill bodies, on the other hand, transform into alternately ethereal and temporal landscapes. Though metaphor's leaps may be swift, for the ill bodies, sensation metastasizes more quickly than description. Language, like medicine, often fails them.

The 1990s were a time of fusion. The fusion trends within music, art, cooking, and academic disciplines seemed to signal a kind of intellectual and creative anarchy in which everyone could diagnose the modern condition, and everyone could heal it. It was a time of taking chances and crossing boundaries. Showalter's reclamation of hysteria—in the age of computer profiling and computer-generated media—capitalized on the cultural fusion of personality, technology, and text, since she tried to spice up classic hysteria by presenting it as a new programming language for the automatons of the modern age. But ironically, it is those bodies that do *not* respond to technology—that elude diagnostic measures, don't heal from technological innovation, and become sick from the fumes of contemporary society—that are seen by people such as Showalter as the most programmable. In this assumption is a strange contradiction used by many narrative diagnosticians, including those from the New Age who say we "create our own reality." The truth is, sick people are not suggestible hypnotics, but rather those with *rebellious* bodies. And Showalter was clutching fast to the golden rule of the new plague years that simply stated, *what we believe will keep us immune.*

Ultimately, she was just one of many people who disruptively blurred the distinction between biology and story. Before CFIDS was even defined as a medical entity, Showalter was blurring these lines. In her 1979 essay titled "Toward a Feminist Poetics," she quoted Florence Nightingale, who suffered for decades with an illness so much like CFIDS that many people have lobbied to rename CFIDS "Nightingale disease." Showalter interpreted Nightingale's plea—"better to have pain than paralysis"—solely as a rebellion against Victorian oppression.[14] It is no wonder that Showalter viewed CFIDS in a similar light, as a hysterical reaction against suburban numbness—and in this, a kind of inept social uprising. "Happily," she later wrote in the same essay, "some recent women's literature . . . has gone beyond reclaiming suffering to its reinvestment."[15] Her similarly literary response to the anguish of CFIDS patients was reminiscent of Marie Antoinette's famous words to the poor, "Let them eat cake," utterly dismissive in the manner of one unfamiliar with such grief.

Showalter, though, wanted everyone to know just how much *she* had suffered—mainly for things such as addressing feminist backlash after admitting her penchant for nice clothes. "A passion for fashion can sometimes seem a shameful secret life . . ." she wrote. "I think it's time I came out of the closet."[16] In her zealous embrace of the psychological cure, Showalter also began to portray herself as a righteous, embattled warrior. Perhaps because she felt victimized by the many detractors who found her academic discipline too vague to succeed in a high-tech economy, Showalter turned her bitter pen against the poorly defined. And, perhaps because she had been subjected to infighting in her ivory-tower world during the "third wave" of feminism, Showalter appropriated some of the more simplistic accoutrements of feminist criticism, such as the use of seemingly irrelevant French phrases like *fin de siècle*, while taking a radically antifeminist turn. It was more than easy for her to capitalize on the pervasive misogyny around CFIDS, an illness still widely attributed to women's excesses ("hysteria" and "overachiever" have a similar root—the assumption that women should not be, do, or feel too much). But what really made Showalter a true *hystorian* by her own definition (a person whose reality is heavily influenced by media narratives) was the fact that she insistently relied on popular magazines, not the numerous respected medical texts full of clinical evidence about CFIDS, to prove her own hysteria theory. Her book cited magazines such as *Newsweek* and *McCall's* as medical evidence. Showalter didn't speak to a single person with CFIDS, stating that one-on-one interviews "are generally considered very bad evidence."[17]

Astonishingly, her credibility was hardly questioned. A segment of *CNN Crossfire* on April 20, 1997, pitted Showalter against Hillary Johnson—a woman who spent almost a decade of her CFIDS years meticulously researching every aspect of her own illness, interviewing over 500 clinicians, politicians, and civilians, with some of the most impressive investigative journalism since Watergate. It should have been like pitting a phrenologist against a brain surgeon. But Johnson was called upon to defend her credibility and prove the factuality of her own diagnosis. Showalter's theory—in contrast—was given surprising merit. The bias of this debate shone a harsh light on how CFIDS has been misrepresented by the media. When Johnson pointed out that Showalter ignored hundreds of CFIDS studies documenting physiological abnormalities, for example, the moderator asked her why she was so "insulted" by the notion of CFIDS being caused by stress or having psychiatric origins. Johnson replied, "If chronic fatigue syndrome were caused by stress or by reading about it in the newspaper, as Elaine Showalter claims in her book, why don't we all have chronic fatigue syndrome?"

"Well, maybe we do," replied the moderator.

"Well, I don't think you do, Lynne," said Johnson, calmly. "Because I don't think you'd be working."

After this apt retort, the moderator questioned how Johnson could have completed her book (in over nine years, mind you) if *she* was really so disabled. I'm sure the same moderator would never have said to Christopher Reeve, the paralyzed actor who played Superman, that he must not really have a spinal cord injury because he was able to direct a film. Johnson, like the rest of us on disability, probably had to compile an enormous amount of medical proof to wear the label "disabled." But sadly, mountains of evidence don't hold weight against visual cues in the era of empiricism. Exasperated at Johnson's insistence in pointing out the obvious, the moderator simply discounted her by quipping: "You seem very energetic."[18]

When people criticized Showalter as an insulated member of the literary elite, she posted to the English grad e-mail list "E-Grad" about how she once spent her paltry graduate teaching fellowship on a sewing machine to sew her own clothes (to prove she was not an ivory-tower academic who had never suffered). She also announced that she had once had a bout with hysteria but had cured herself. In *Harper's Magazine,* she said CFIDS patients were giving her death threats as she embarked on a book tour ("Bullets are too good for you!" shouted one at her reading). She described her audiences—disgruntled CFIDS patients, conspiracy theorists, and a 400-pound alien abductee from the Bronx who "didn't know there were aliens in the hood." She even took a moment to parody the power of metaphor, describing an abductee who said aliens helped him to realize that he kept urinating on his girlfriend because he was "pissed off at her." Showalter concluded the *Harper's* piece with a joke about the rabid CFIDS activists who were trying to kill her: "In retrospect, their death threats seem comic and oxymoronic: if a tired person had actually summoned up the energy to assassinate me, we would have been the number-one joke on Leno and Letterman for a week."[19]

Perhaps CFIDS patients could have laughed at this if Showalter weren't perpetrating another form of strange hysteria, the hysteria of people who have read a few bad articles about CFIDS and claimed to be experts on a complex disorder, trumpeting their strange and insistent ideas wherever possible. Psychologist Katrina Berne, PhD, described Showalter's scholarship this way: "When you give a 5-year-old a hammer, everything starts to look like a nail."[20] *Hystories* garnered more media attention than any CFIDS medical book and advanced

Showalter's career. Though it had very real consequences for millions of patients who are often told by doctors they are crazy, Showalter was not censured by Princeton for her poor scholarship. She simply couldn't understand why her book angered CFIDS patients. "It's not a question of insurance and disability, which they're getting,"[21] she wrote, though in fact CFIDS patients are only half as likely as those with other disabilities to garner benefits on initial applications.[22] On the other hand, Showalter's book was followed by her prestigious appointment as president of the Modern Languages Association.

My friend once joked, "Well, if it's *fin de siècle* panic, as Showalter says, at least you should recover soon after the turn of the millennium." But meanwhile, I can sometimes empathize with the despair of patient David Hinds, who wrote, "Wait for the millennium? I'm going down to the local tavern right now to hoist a few to the memory of the healthy person I'll never be again."[23]

THE PROBLEM WITH METAPHOR AND ILLNESS

Showalter preached an antidote of "dedication and persistence" to cure hysterical epidemics (after all, if one's symptoms are metaphorical, one should be able to think them away).[24] This notion was hardly original. Hysteria is a very old concept, and "cures" for hysteria have often been as metaphorical as the diagnosis itself. Many contemporary beliefs about immunity have also been scripted through metaphor. The same people who chose purebred dogs for their personality traits or lack of predisposition toward hip dysplasia bought pop psychology books by the dozen in the 1990s, believing in the "power of the mind" to change emotion and illness. Capitalist ideals infiltrated new economies, heralding a triumph of individualism that became characterized in America by fitness guru infomercials and talk show hosts motivating people to change their personalities and bodies. As a consequence, people rebelled against any notions of genetic determinism, talking loudly about the correlation between behavior and disease and staging personal warfare on bacteria and germs. In an emerging climate of self-diagnosis, self-prevention, and self-cure, narrative became a means of controlling the body. Nevertheless, illness (not anyone's chosen story) remained, as Anatole Broyard wrote, "a kind of incoherence,"[25] and incoherence has always been the first target of metaphoric exploration.

Many writers have elucidated the problems of viewing illness metaphorically, asserting that illness lives outside of its cognition, in the realm of pure sensation. Others have pointed out that much of our cultural understanding of illness stems from metaphors, derived from science, or shamanism. But metaphor is part of the finite scrawls of fiction and poetry. Chronic illness, on the other hand, is a baffling story that does not necessarily end. The real story of illness is only communicable through minute, microscopic transmission, through pathogens and not words. Metaphor, though it is descriptive, is not in itself diagnostic. Rather, metaphor is transportational—or, as Robert Bly speaks of it in *Leaping Poetry*—a means of taking leaps; leaps of faith, leaps of knowledge, leaps between conscious and subconscious states.[26] It is a catapult away from language and an attempt at unification between language and the elusive world beyond it.

According to the poet Federico Garcia Lorca, metaphor should not be a mere substitution for visceral experience—an insertion of a word such as *hysteria* to describe mysterious expression—but a reckoning with death itself, inherently physical, an extension of the flesh and the spirit. Lorca writes that all good metaphor must possess *duende,* a divine energy that comes from the awareness of death in life and pushes one to live passionately. Metaphor, if used in this way, could fill in the gaps of empirical thinking and expand our knowledge of the mysteries of the body. "Intelligence is often the enemy of poetry," Lorca writes. "It elevates the poet to a sharp-edged throne where he forgets that ants could eat him or that a great arsenic lobster could fall suddenly on his head."[27] His argument is that art—which promotes understanding and empathy—must lie outside of immunity myths. "With *duende,*" he writes, "it is easier to love and understand."[28] Lorca's fearless vision of art and metaphor, one that embraces the realities of the body and its inevitable failings, is distinctly different from the constructions of metaphor many have used to build a card house of seeming immunity against the ill.

German poet Rainer Maria Rilke also had a sense of this *duende* logic. According to one critic, Rilke saw writing poetry as "a reverie on the inexplicable image of a cup balancing on the level back of a hand. He saw that cup filled with a pure liquid, a blue distillation, which he understood to be an extract of death itself." The characters in the poem "seem to go on living only because they are afraid of drinking the poisonous liquid" and thus "the poem sputters down into an incomprehensible mumbling."[29] In other words, illness and metaphor are close cousins, in a sense removed from science, which tries to fend off the body's decline. Metaphor cannot be used by the healthy to diagnose the sick, if used with empirical remoteness, because the healthy must touch death before understanding metaphors of illness—and even then, good metaphor itself is not a tonic, but a true expedition into the realm of the ill. This is where metaphor has failed the scribes of sick populations, who have assumed that not only empathy, but a brand of medicine born out of the magical thinking of the immune, can be reached through metaphor alone.

If metaphor is transportational, it can also be reckless and catastrophic. It has been twenty years since Susan Sontag wrote the line "Illness is not a metaphor."[30] Yet the public has increasingly turned to metaphors to transport them from the parameters of medicine. In a century when mind-body medicine has emerged as the mantra for the new millennium, when the body has become a subject of discourse in literary theory and legal ethics, many have been seduced into using metaphor's vehicular powers to bridge the gap between description and pure sensation. In the midst of millennial epidemiological panic, the metaphors surrounding chronic fatigue syndrome have become a true bandwagon, an insular bus through the quarantine zone.

Of course, metaphors can be effective communication tools, even in the universe of quick-fix managed medicine. A patient walks into a doctor's office and offers a tale of her disintegration. The patient and doctor stand in the borderlands of their separate physical knowledge, offering halting translations. These stories form a flawed oral tradition, often based on a parable logic in which heroic archetypes—in this case, physicians—convey the rationale of inexplicable pain. The problem is this: there is no universal language between the sick and the well. We reside in different countries, between which there is a river of forgetfulness, a Lethe. We cannot necessarily know each other. We are more *unlike* than like.

As I said before, in the wrath of illness, empiricism is most certainly the hurricane's eye. *Duende* metaphors—metaphors that really touch the visceral human experience—require being in touch with the hurricane. As Charlotte Joko Beck writes in *Nothing Special: Living Zen,* human nature tries to find calm in the heart of destruction. Many of the metaphors used for illness are ways of asserting that calm, asserting distance. Beck tells a story of a commercial pilot and a hang glider, both caught in the winds of a hurricane. The pilot, with the illusion of control, desperately steers for the eye of the storm. He is like most of us—forever seeking stability in the tumult of life. The hang glider, however, has lost what Helen Keller called the "superstition" of security, and thus he decides to simply have the ride of his life. Both men come to the same end in this story. Both men die.[31] But like Helen Keller, people with CFIDS have had superstition stolen from us. We do not necessarily believe that the almighty eye of medicine, or the engine power of metaphor, can save us. Our bodies are a constant lesson in mortality. We've got to navigate the wind.

THE SATIRISTS

Hillary Johnson, in *Osler's Web,* writes compellingly of the way government officials turned an epidemic into an acceptable social parody. Gary Holmes, one of the two government researchers sent to examine the famous Incline Village outbreak of the illness, responded to criticism about his affiliation with CFIDS by filling his office with a series of CFIDS parodies. On his door, he posted a fake letter composed by agency staff, a letter that depicted a malingerer turning to the CDC for help. "Dear Sirs," it read. "I am sick . . . I am so tired." At this point, the satirical subject waxed hypochondriacal, stating, in part, "I would like a list of recommended treatments . . . in descending order of trendiness, including . . . sensory deprivation, walking on hot coals, alternating sensory deprivation and walking on hot coals, purified fruit-bat guano injections, and bedrest." Then he asked for information on obtaining disability benefits for his "disease."[32]

Many humorists began depicting the diagnosis as culturally symbolic in an age of exhaustion, a vague ailment that anyone could pretend to have. Woody Allen took a moment in his film *Deconstructing Harry* to portray his famous hypochondriac persona spouting off a list of imagined chic ailments, including chronic fatigue syndrome. The 1999 movie *Mumford,* about a man in a small town pretending to be a therapist, approached the hypochondria angle again. Actress Hope

Davis played Sophie Crisp, a young divorcée with chronic fatigue syndrome. "She's so depressed that she's become ill with chronic fatigue syndrome or Epstein-Barr virus, or whatever," said Davis in the Touchtone Pictures production notes. With method acting ingenuity, Davis even wore lead weights in her shoes to feel dragged down. Dr. Mumford prescribed a program of walking exercises for Sophie, during which she talked to him about her postdivorce ennui and her bickering mother, which eventually led to a full recovery.[33] The film added to the growing cultural metaphor of CFIDS as a "whatever" kind of illness, a malaise that could simply be walked off.

This notion permeated all media. The cartoon *Kudzu,* which is syndicated in major newspapers such as *The Boston Globe* and *The Washington Post,* did two strips mocking CFIDS, even after negative response to the first one, which treated CFIDS as a form of social meteorology. "We have that chronic fatigue syndrome moving into the area . . . with an eighty percent chance of lethargy and lack of motivation today and tonight," wrote the cartoonist. "The forecast for tomorrow: vague!"[34] It suddenly seemed as though CFIDS could be used as a catchall metaphor—one that could even be exploited in advertising campaigns. A billboard in Australia, erected at the Sydney airport for the 2000 Olympic crowd, promoted a vacation spot by depicting a lazy couple floating down an aquamarine channel in a rowboat, with a banner headline that simply read, "chronic fatigue syndrome," and then the trailer, "Hamilton. The island that's spoiling Australia." The billboard perpetuated the common myth that CFIDS is just one long vacation.

The acceptability of CFIDS parodies was astonishingly widespread. My friend, who was so debilitated by CFIDS and multiple chemical sensitivities that she traveled with an oxygen tank, received a humorous greeting card one day. The card—produced by Carlton Cards (a subsidiary of American Greetings)—began with a cartoon drawing of a frazzled-looking woman. "Sorry I haven't written!" The front cover exclaimed. On the inside it said, "But I came down with a bad case of chronic fatigue syndrome, and it's been really hard to find the ti . . ." (the word trailed off into a bunch of sleepy "zzzzzz's" at the bottom of the page).[35] Mocking arthritis or multiple sclerosis or lupus this way would be considered appalling, but the CFIDS ridicule seemed oddly accepted.

Television shows jumped on the lampoon bandwagon. On the Fox network's animated show *King of the Hill,* a character "pretended" to have chronic fatigue syndrome so she could demand workplace accommodations, then sprawled on the office couch all day. On October 24, 1999, the same night that CNN aired a persuasive special about CFIDS, a character on the legendary animated show *The Simpsons* joked about CFIDS, saying that it belonged in the "chick stuff" section of a newspaper. Later, Al Franken wrote a "humorous" book called *Why Not Me?* in which he described what the world would be like if the president pretended to have CFIDS. Magazines such as *OUT* depicted it as a trendy disease that anyone could use to "deny all allegations, claiming that chronic fatigue syndrome prevents you from writing anything but your signature."[36] Previously, papers around the country mockingly threw about the coinage "yuppie flu" to describe the affluent, white sufferers who were first diagnosed in Incline Village, Nevada, in the early 1980s. CFIDS, like disco, came to be seen as a pathetic, maligned ideology that could be burned like bad 1970s vinyl.

The hostility toward yuppies that grew in the counterculture of the 1980s, with such sentiments as "kill yuppie scum," quickly carried over to those suffering from this strange malady. CFIDS was not seen as a legitimate pathology, but as a pathological ideology—a label embraced by those who wanted an excuse for their bourgeois exhaustion. Indeed, in the cure-driven frenzy of managed medicine, chronic fatigue syndrome was just a triad of inexact and potentially limitless (read: unmanageable) words—in effect, a set of symbols about as palpable to the public as obesity. The public grabbed this poorly defined nomenclature and quickly placed the blame on the victims.

THE ETYMOLOGISTS

But chronic fatigue syndrome appears to be a simpler story than it is. Something as simple as fatigue, like snow to an Inuit, may have hundreds of variations in its insular population. A feminist critic rattling off a few French words, or a New Age guru prescribing a Native American herbal cure, is usually just a sequestered Californian trying to comprehend Inuit snow. But in the era of managed care, nonspecific language affects the marketing and the subsequent funding for an illness. As Mary Schweitzer put it: "The name 'chronic fatigue syndrome' presents an immense rhetorical advantage to insurance companies, and a similarly immense rhetorical disadvantage to patients, just because it means, 'tired all the time and unwilling to suck it up like the rest of us do.' "[37] Indeed, early on in the CFIDS struggle, insurance companies began setting limitations around "fatigue-related conditions," though I doubt they meant heart disease or postchemotherapy fatigue.

Though a name-change debate has raged for years in the CFIDS community, and most researchers have argued that a new name should be based on a clinical marker, the naming of illness is more an art than a science, almost poetic in nature. Cancer comes from the Greek *karkinos* and Latin *cancer,* both meaning crab, to describe the crablike appearance of the veins in external tumors. Lupus is named after the Latin word for wolf, because of the characteristic malar rash that develops on the face, giving sufferers a wolflike appearance. Multiple sclerosis is named after the hardened tissue that forms patches in the brain and spinal cord. Herpes comes from the Greek and means to "creep like a serpent." Syphilis was named for a hero of a sixteenth-century poem. Influenza, formerly named grippe after the French word for seizure, was renamed after the Italian word for influence, based upon the belief that epidemics are influenced by the stars. Lyme disease is named after a town in Connecticut. Yellow fever is named after the color it turns its victims.[38]

Though sophisticated tests pinpoint numerous physiological abnormalities in patients, CFIDS has been depicted as amorphous and, instead of being given a poetic name to render the felt quality of the symptoms, named after a concept so pedestrian it has been drained of meaning. "Fatigue" is a nondescript word. Like "depression," it is a word most people think they have experienced. But while the difference between rainy-day sadness and suicidal depression is huge, so is the gap between standard tiredness and CFIDS fatigue. People with CFIDS often have trouble walking between rooms or lifting a grocery bag. The illness produces complete bodily catastrophe.

Gary Holmes, the same man who mocked CFIDS in his own government office, is the one who proposed the name chronic fatigue syndrome.[39] This fact reeks of an almost blatant government conspiracy to keep sufferers, as Hillary Johnson writes, "in a Kafkaesque universe where what they knew to be real was reported by authorities to be patently false."[40] The government has dragged its feet for years on the name-change issue. The damage of the name has been tremendous, damage that will take many years to correct even after a new name is adopted.

The notion of CFIDS as a vague condition simply arose out of its vague terminology. Charles Darwin, when he first heard a description of a giraffe, exclaimed, "There cannot be such an animal."[41] CFIDS, even bigger than a medical giraffe, is almost like *Sesame Street*'s elusive giant puppet Snuffleupagus—witnessed only by believers. A study titled "Stigma and Chronic Fatigue Syndrome" found that more than 75 percent of CFIDS patients have been labeled a psychological case by at least one physician. Most of these seek out other doctors, leading to a self-perpetuating cycle in which disbelieving doctors rarely see progressive cases of CFIDS.[42] Doctors who see many patients with CFIDS say that its symptoms are not comparable, that false cases are easy to pick out, and that "there is no disease even vaguely like it."[43] Because of the lack of funding for physician education, most doctors are not even aware of the strict CDC guidelines for CFIDS diagnosis. Generally, people with CFIDS experience some combination of debilitating symptoms every single day. For diagnosis, symptoms must be so severe as to cause a significant reduction of activity over an extended period (a level could be objectively measured, according to the researcher Pascale De Becker, through bicycle exercise tests that show decreased performance ability).[44] The symptoms are not vague. They are merely so grand and evasive that, like the elephantine Snuffleupagus, they require a perceptive witness.

The New Age response to CFIDS has demonstrated how simplistic metaphors can be derived from a name, then used to exploit and shame an illness population. When I confessed how desperately ill I actually was to a reiki healer, she mentioned she was a student of Louise Hay and firmly believed people choose to be sick. New Age gurus such as Hay have made a killing off of metaphoric diagnosis. Hay's book, *You Can Heal Your Life,* equates simplistic metaphors to symptoms. It is not hard to come up with a metaphor of "inability to see ahead with joy" for cataracts. It doesn't take a poetic genius to come up with the metaphor of "a refusal to change" for chronic disease. For CFIDS (which she seems to categorize under chronic Epstein-Barr virus, one former name for the illness), Hay tells patients they are pushing beyond their limits, afraid of "not being good enough," and "draining all inner support." Indeed, these metaphors became pervasive symbols early on in the CFIDS struggle.[45]

But most of Hay's observations are based on the notion of fatigue, not chronic fatigue syndrome. "Chronic fatigue" is a symptom of a number of illnesses besides CFIDS. Still, "chronic fatigue" or simply "fatigue" quickly became popularized shorthand for CFIDS, even on medical records, though these terms represented only one symptom of the whole complex. Imagine such inaccurate and derogatory descriptors carrying over into other illnesses, how ludicrous it would sound, for example, if posttracheotomy patients were said to have "chronic mime syndrome." The word "fatigue" seemed to provoke about as much enthusiasm as the word "mime," and CFIDS was viewed as an acquired identity, a kind of annoying, suburban whiteface. But it wasn't that. It was more like a hidden mountain on a day of thick cloud cover, something immense but unseen.

MY OWN PRIVATE EVEREST

I was in continual agony; I have never in my whole life been so tired.

alpinist Reinhold Messner,
about the first ascent of Mount Everest
completed without supplemental oxygen[46]

When I read Jon Krakauer's famous account of the tragic cluster of Mount Everest fatalities, *Into Thin Air,* I marveled at the descriptions of survivors at the highest-altitude camp after they returned from their summit push. For me, CFIDS has often felt like Krakauer's descriptions of altitude sickness, hypoxic dementia, and profound exhaustion. With the impaired brain blood flow CFIDS patients experience, the conditions may be more analogous than science has begun to ponder.[47] Numerous other CFIDS sufferers—including one who scaled many peaks and scuba dived extensively before getting sick—have agreed with me that the symptoms of CFIDS, including the fatigue, resemble an improbably chronic hypoxic state, so far from normal tiredness, so much more of an all-body impairment, than the word fatigue could ever convey. As Chris Norris wrote in *New York Magazine,* "If this is fatigue, its relationship to workaday weariness is as Sartre's nausea was to an upset tummy. I have been tired before. This is not tired."[48] Many of the Everest survivors in Krakauer's book were fumbling around in utter confusion, unable to cross the smallest distance without grave difficulty. Many of them were so exhausted they literally could not move from their sleeping bags. This type of exhaustion, fatigue combined with profound brain dysfunction and a feeling that the body is depleted on a deep cellular level, is perhaps a little like the exhaustion CFIDS patients talk about. As Patti Skari, the former alpinist and diver, described: "One of my friends climbed Annapurna. He told me how he would put one foot up and take about ten breaths, plod the other foot higher and take about ten breaths. That sounds like me climbing the stairs to my apartment."[49] This is why the semantics of the word fatigue are so important.

Unlike the survivors of Everest, people with CFIDS are still trying to prove that there ever was, or is, an Everest. Like children in a dysfunctional household, we are told by many in the medical community (and most in the metaphor community) that the mountain in our midst is indeed just a molehill. I believe this happens because distance is a reductionistic tool, and most people who have spoken out loudly against CFIDS have had little contact with actual patients. Even when one woman offered Elaine Showalter "a pint of my A-negative blood anytime she wants to demonstrate to herself her conviction that my disease is *fin de siècle* angst,"[50] Showalter was not interested in a pure interpretation *or* a transfusion. Government "experts" on CFIDS employed the same approach, using their trips to the first outbreak in the ski town of Incline Village as sightseeing vacations and barely seeing patients. Generally, those approaching from such a distance—employing the transportational power of metaphor—could deny all depth perception by simply pinching their fingers together at arm's length and scaling down the distant mountain in front of them.

Like most metaphoric fables gone mad, CFIDS has become an urban legend. The narratives of the actual patients have been subsumed under a strange set of myths that have nothing to do with the actual illness experience. The Elaine Showalters and Louise Hays have become the misinformed voices of the sick.

Most troubling to CFIDS patients is the fact that our daily heroics—like our invisible Everest and diminishing fingerprints—are undetectable to the common eye. Often, the heroics of CFIDS involve profound deprivation and restriction—forcing ourselves to not do things that matter to us, resting a week just to go to the grocery store. As a society, we have all seen the image of the paraplegic with his arms braced as he slowly makes his way across parallel bars in a courageous attempt at physical therapy. But CFIDS heroics are different from that. To truly witness them requires a *duende* metaphor, almost blind faith.

In fact, when the CFIDS community did produce a hero of sorts—soccer player Michelle Akers, who became a hero not only when she helped lead the U.S. Women's Soccer team to its World Cup Victory in 1999, but also when she spoke openly and courageously about her battle with CFIDS—her effect on all of us was mixed. As a woman so strong she could not possibly be called hysterical, she called into question everything we know about disability. As a mild case of CFIDS (though she was virtually bedridden in the early stages), she also called into question everything CFIDS patients knew about their own experience. Michelle herself oozes resilience and determination from every pore. I love her unflinching honesty and courage. Unshakable and charming, Michelle has gone an extra 10,000 miles to prove that CFIDS is not a disease of the faint of heart. In front of Congress, on behalf of many others and myself, she explained the paradox of CFIDS: "The harder you work, the more it drags you down. The more it disables you."[51] Nobody could better make such a powerful statement to refute the oppressive idiocy of behaviorists and "holistic" medicine gurus such as Dr. Andrew Weil, who insistently encourage those with CFIDS to just exercise more. Michelle has no qualms about being forthright and showing that disability is not shameful. She demonstrates that CFIDS—like all illnesses—occurs on a spectrum, that disability can be astoundingly invisible and complex. After her team's World Cup victory, the team doctor stated, "It wasn't that other players didn't suffer to stay at the top. It was take that and multiply it by ten for Michelle."[52] Michelle—one of the top athletes in the world—must have IVs put in at halftime, stay on an unbelievably strict diet, forgo product endorsements because she doesn't have the energy to make public appearances, and have her teammates carry her bags at the airport. Plus, she must spend her nonpractice time resting—not accompanying her teammates to Disney World, not following them to the White House for a personal speech from the president. Yet, while people can easily accept that a disabled wheelchair racer is suffering, though he might not feel *sick* most of the time, they cannot accept that Michelle Akers—who suffers minute by minute with excruciating symptoms—is disabled. Michelle has an atypical case of CFIDS—since most patients suffer extreme exercise intolerance and grow progressively worse after any mild exertion—but she does suffer, a lot.

And though such stories should perhaps provide grounds for empathy, they often inadvertently shame those stories of disability that lack made-for-TV drama, stories in which perseverance over daily agony is not glamorous or dramatic but tragically mundane. The healthy—more often than the sick—tell stories of disabled heroics, nicely parceled tales that are designed to incite careful compassion but to avoid the fear that narrative itself is contagious. The real stories of disability—like the meandering tales of too many veterans—seem to present an intolerable pacing. On the contrary, images of quick heroism perpetuate the notion that if you grin, if you push, you can persevere. And really, the quest for cultural heroes in the face of disability poses the question wrong. As Camus writes in *The Plague,* "There's no question of heroism in all this. It's a matter of common decency."[53]

THE CULTURAL HISTORY OF AN EPIDEMIC

Chronic fatigue syndrome became part of the hip new iconography of social satirists, symbolism for an overworked age, the embodiment of a neurotic society trying to laugh at itself—a postmodern dumb blonde joke. But how, and why, could so many people get away with mocking a group of desperately ill people? Many social trends contributed to this corruption of common decency. As an invisible disability in an era of skepticism, CFIDS posed an interesting cultural challenge. The early images of yuppie flu, which portrayed mostly affluent white women as being ill, emerged just as political correctness was taking over America. As difference became the catchword on campus, disenfranchised groups struggled for team recognition. With this struggle came visual markers of race, class, sexuality. Individuals began to display their affiliations to groups. And while the word invisibility was bantered about, visible displays of oppression and uprising—the ACT UP activists throwing blood at the White House, Earth First members chaining themselves to trees—became public images of group affiliation and cultural fragmentation.

Disability was also portrayed with an increasingly visible symbol—the stick figure in a wheelchair. With the emergence of such visual symbolism, however, came a hostility and distrust of the invisible and subclinical. With the need for affiliation came an almost obsessive need to categorize. There was simply no room, in this era, for the emergence of an invisible epidemic, one that rarely displayed itself on the patients' faces and often eluded basic blood tests. CFIDS was an illness of translation, not affiliation, one that baffled technology and time.

It cannot be underestimated how much AIDS politics both eclipsed and influenced the lives of CFIDS patients. Many writers have also pointed out bizarre and alarming connections between the two illnesses—such as similarities in brain scans and elevated HHV-6 titers. Dr. Paul Cheney, though, noticed what is perhaps the most remarkable correlative. When he entered data for 400 CFIDS patients into a computer, noting their time of onset and other factors, he found that CFIDS and AIDS cases have occurred—over time—at almost parallel rates of growth.[54] But AIDS medical psychology also dramatically affected CFIDS patients. In the rhetoric of the AIDS years, people were taught to view illness as an outcome of behavior. Every illness in this era was shaped by the furor of AIDS politics. Even Showalter talked about CFIDS and Gulf War syndrome as "sickness lifestyles."[55] This description was not unlike the homophobic AIDS rhetoric that confused gay "lifestyle" with susceptibility. Once contagion was equated with behavior, and identity politics took over, pairing of illness and identity was almost inevitable. A strange contradiction emerged in this era when words such as "multiculturalism" entered the public arena—the need to *identify,* along with the need to believe in the transcendence of inborn identity.

AIDS politics embodied this new contradiction. As Simon LeVay tried to prove that gayness was a genetic identity (a notion that some gay groups embraced, and others saw as dangerous), gay-dominated AIDS activist groups explored the notion that AIDS began as an attempt at genocide, uncovering statistics that an unusually high percentage of the men who took part in government-promoted hepatitis inoculations in New York City later tested HIV positive. Some groups, often including the growing populations of African Americans and Latinos with the virus, explored the notion that HIV was a form of biological terrorism against civilians. Many pointed out that government attempts to prove that AIDS originated in Africa, in apes that fraternized with humans, were based on disturbing presumptions of American racism.[56] Unfortunately, such genocide arguments often provided more fodder for those who would turn identity against the identified. But, when the distinction was blurred between illness and "lifestyle," a tactic that was too often presented by Right Wing extremists who wanted to prove that God created AIDS to purge the world of immorality, these same groups could only revert to a deterministic argument and assert that illness would select who it chose to select.

AIDS proved that the discussion about behavior and illness is a very complicated one. As Michael Callen, the controversial gay author of the book *Surviving AIDS,* asserted, gay men's bathhouses in the late 1970s could very well have been an epidemiological breeding ground.[57] Unfortunately, gay men with AIDS (and later on, drug users and others) were retroactively damned for unknowingly participating in some of the high-risk behaviors that led to HIV infection. AIDS, like the polio epidemic earlier in the century, made people disillusioned with medicine and obsessed with pseudoscience and self-control. Behaviorists desperately looked for qualities that would characterize the "long-term survivor" of HIV and AIDS. Science could not explain why some survived and some perished, so many survivors boiled it down to this dictum of the magical thinkers: "Some said macrobiotics, some said Classic Coke, some said God, some said acupuncture, some said lipids. All said hope."[58] There is nothing wrong with hope, of course, but who *doesn't* hold onto hope until the very end? Louise Hay also began to lead popular seminars for people who were HIV positive. People started to use condoms and clean needles. So, when researchers finally created the drug cocktails that controlled the HIV virus, heralding them as a miracle treatment, the self-deterministic majority believed themselves to play an important role in the triumph of the medical system. These participants in the war on AIDS were not unlike domestic munitions workers in the two world wars who thought themselves to have played an integral role in victory.

THE WAR OF METAPHOR

In fact, I would argue that the cultural climate after the worst stages of a terrifying plague such as AIDS or polio often mimics postwar nationalism. Still in the clutches of a blame-the-enemy mindset, society often enters into an epidemiological cold war of prevention tactics. This period is a war of metaphor, a figurative war that intends to protect against, or simply replicate, real combat. Those who remain ill or disabled are either eventually viewed as forgotten casualties (whose rants on the war years seem paranoid and outdated) or as psychosomatic antinationalist traitors (not unlike the Vietnam vets suffering from post-traumatic stress disorder). When propaganda has claimed that medicine is triumphant, these insistently ill are seen to have weak or even McCarthyist characters. Thus, the mantra of reducing risk factors, propagated by the healthy, does not fade out when a treatment is found. Instead, these plague survivors tend to model themselves after heroes of super-cleanliness, who will prevent further contagion, and also to possess a feeling of superiority over those who have succumbed to illness. In this paradigm, the chronically ill are seen as weak, clingy, and hungry for attention when they are visible, and suspicious when their symptoms are unseen.

After the 1953 discovery of the polio vaccine by Dr. Jonas Salk, and likewise after the invention of protease inhibitors, a model of cleanliness based on self-responsibility rose in popularity. The postpolio model of 1950s motherhood, typified by obsessive domestic cleanliness, reemerged in a new form in the post-AIDS years in the marketing of ubiquitous antibacterial products. Despite the fact that scientists quickly determined these products would lead to strains of super-resistant pathogens, they were snatched up with a paranoid fervor. Commercials showed the perils of independence and personal responsibility, represented by the man at the dirty ATM machine who didn't treat his hands with Purell, and the consequences of not practicing prevention, exemplified by the mother who didn't wipe her child's germ-covered apple with an antibacterial paper towel. The Good Mother in all of us, in the years of self-parenting, would protect the suburbs from the ills of modern society—dirty sex, dirty money, the dirty bus terminals of sprawling cities. We would be rid of weakness and genetic inferiority. And, it should not be overlooked that in the safer sex era, the word *cleanliness* became commonly associated with the disturbing language of genocide, with the term *ethnic cleansing.*

Just as women were assigned to domestic jobs that would help efforts of the world wars, in postplague years the Good Mother of cleanliness has carried out the common law of organized society. The Good Mother, like the Good Slave, is a cultural model of complicity. Her job is to justify the violence that just took place to pretend we are all part of the same victorious front. Just as antiracist racists would argue that Good Slaves love their work, and are therefore not oppressed, antifeminist feminists might argue that Rosie the Riveter or June Cleaver are the truly liberated women, happily building war planes and baking unnaturally white cakes. The post-protease inhibitor years were thus the perfect time for Showalter's hysteria argument. After all, what is a hysteric but a Bad Mother, a woman who can't take responsibility or get a grip. But illness is not a behavior or a lifestyle choice. Just as ex-gay ministries cannot "cure" gays, neither can the New Hysterians or the New Age banish all diseases by force of will.

In an era that witnessed the fall of Eastern Europe, the reconfiguring of the family system, and the profound devastation of AIDS, many approached the millennium with an apocalyptic fervor and a sense of living amid global fragmentation. CFIDS, a multisystemic disrupter with no clear cause, might have been construed as symbolic of these cultural changes, and it left people scrambling for explanation. This explanation came, most conveniently, in the form of metaphor, stereotype, and conjecture. A society of intense intermingling felt too out of control to various conservative reactionaries who feared cultural diversity and loss of authority, and this kind of society existed *within* the bodies of CFIDS patients, a world where any part of the body could seemingly be targeted, where no part seemed particularly immune. I believe CFIDS patients became a metaphor for cultural vagueness, and ultimately, implosion. Already scorned by liberals who wanted to bury the Republican years and their yuppie credo, people with CFIDS were now condemned by conservatives afraid of a new, inclusive democracy.

Perhaps some form of *fin de siècle* panic did arise in the 1980s and 1990s. In my opinion, however, this panic was a mass fear of being left behind, like the CFIDS victims, in a world spinning too quickly into the next millennium, and a fear about autonomous survival in the midst of cultural cross-pollination. Once President Clinton spun tales of a visionary society that would embrace difference (never mind that one of his greatest failures was his unsuccessful attempt to implement national health care), the American Dream was revived in a new form, a form that proposed opportunity for all Americans with sufficient drive and a certain degree of flexibility. CFIDS thus became culturally symbolic of all those who could not *Just Do It* at whim—i.e., the ones who weren't trying hard enough. Simultaneously, a strange sort of figure started to take over in lieu of the yuppie. This prototype was able to maneuver Web sites, swill microbrewery beer, get Tantric, and go ice climbing on the weekends—his body was technologically adept and physically invincible, a model for the future. And anybody who was disabled by the fast-paced world, well, they'd better just get over it, because the millennium would not wait for them.

MOMENTARY VISIBILITY
AND PRIVATE HARM

Though a public mythology surrounds CFIDS, the patient population remains largely private and unnoticed. Although Showalter mentions that she has gotten regular e-mail insults from CFIDS sufferers, contending that e-mail must be a "safe and irresistible outlet" for patients,[59] she doesn't realize that most people with the illness are largely homebound. The networks are quite hidden, not because of subversion, as Showalter seems to think, but because of symptomatology. Plus, people with CFIDS tend to "pass" in the outside world. Few of us appear to be as sick as we are. Since so few people understand how profoundly debilitating the illness is, social mythology undermines communication of the private, profound suffering CFIDS patients go through.

In group process theory, a subject who returns to the collective after an absence and vaguely says he was sick, without explanation or apology, will tend to be shunned by the rest of the members, who assume abandonment, concoct paranoid motives, and distrust the person's honesty. Because so many people with CFIDS simply disappear from the social fabric, deprived of an accurate language for their condition, they are often shunned by the people around them. Many of my own friends, like a herd of prey animals leaving behind the lame, disappeared in a sea of miscommunication when I got sick. I had no way of talking about what was happening, not only because I developed language-retrieval problems, but because there was no accurate symptomatic vocabulary. Uninsured and undiagnosed, my experience was incomprehensible to me. I became incommunicado, and many people did simply assume the worst, approaching me with suspicion, refusing to utter the name of my diagnosis, and experiencing shame, along with me, for standing up for my rights in public. This illness does not befit exhibitionistic martyrs, as some might think. It is generally, rather, a lonely and private agony.

What Showalter portrays as an aggressive patient movement is simply a group of desperately ill people protecting themselves against real dangers. The *CFIDS Chronicle* surveyed its readership and found that 54 percent of respondents had been sick for more than five years. Most of the survey respondents had sampled numerous treatments—allopathic and alternative. Sadly, many of the only available treatments for CFIDS, and the most commonly prescribed, caused "harmful" results in 20 percent or more of those who tried them.[60] Also, traveling to appointments and shelling out extra cash are often so exhaustive of patients' resources that they depart after just a few treatments, leading some practitioners to believe they must be cured. One patient, who was featured in his local newspaper, was bombarded by pseudocures after the article on his illness appeared. "I received a deluge of telephone and mail solicitations for alternative medicine products, treatments and clinics, and multiple testimonials and anecdotes of miraculous cures," he wrote in a letter to the *Chronicle*. "Most had a substantial price, and the majority involved multi-level marketing."[61]

Fundamentally, science begins with an assumption. If this assumption is infallibility, impossibility, or irritation, then the illness at hand will never be cured. Most people with CFIDS don't want their illness glamorized; they merely want the public to understand its relentless debilitation. Although certain metaphors of illness may appeal to romantics, or escapists, people with CFIDS need a vehicle that accommodates their bodies and transports them toward potential recovery, or at least toward hope. The beauty of metaphor is that it can convey the unspeakable, that which exists on the foggy horizon of articulation. I do believe, as Broyard writes, that metaphor also has the power to be a kind of "literary aspirin."[62] People with CFIDS would love to see their suffering articulated accurately, so they can leave that foggy horizon temporarily, and thus move back to the center of their own lives.

NOTES

1. Ostrom, Neenyah. *America's Biggest Cover-Up: 50 More Things Everyone Should Know About the Chronic Fatigue Syndrome Epidemic and Its Link to AIDS.* New York: TNM, Inc., 1993, p. 52.

2. Ehrlich, George E. Book Review. "Chronic Fatigue and Its Syndromes," by Simon Wessely, Matthew Hotopf, and Michael Sharpe. *Journal of the American Medical Association, 282*(11), September 15, 1999, p. 1093.

3. Stenger, Victor. "Postmodern Attacks on Science and Reality." (From the Web site: <www.Quackwatch.com>.)

4. Carpman, Vicki. "New Book Perpetuates Myth of CFIDS As Hysteria." *The CFIDS Chronicle,* Spring 1997. Quote is from Marsha T. Wallace, pp. 6-9.

5. Travis, Carol. "Pursued by Fashionable Furies." *The New York Times Book Review,* May 4, 1997, p. 28.

6. Showalter, Elaine. *Hystories: Hysterical Epidemics and Modern Media.* New York: Columbia University Press, 1997, p. 4.

7. Ibid., p. 6.

8. Ibid., p. 7.

9. Ibid., p. 10.

10. Ibid., p. 7.

11. Ehrlich, George E. Book Review. "Chronic Fatigue and Its Syndromes."

12. Carpman, "New Book Perpetuates Myth."

13. Carr, C. "The Hysterian Meets the Chronically Fatigued: Truth or Consequences." *The Village Voice,* May 20, 1997, p. 50.

14. Showalter, Elaine. "Toward a Feminist Poetics." In *The New Feminist Criticism,* ed. Elaine Showalter. New York: Pantheon, 1985, p. 133.

15. Ibid., p. 138.

16. Eakin, Emily. "Who's Afraid of Elaine Showalter?" *Lingua Franca,* September 1998, p. 29.

17. Carr, "The Hysterian Meets the Chronically Fatigued."

18. Cheney, Lynne with Elaine Showalter and Hillary Johnson. *CNN Crossfire Sunday,* April 20, 1997.

19. Showalter, Elaine. "Chronic Publicity Syndrome." *Harper's Magazine,* July 1998, pp. 27-30.

20. Carpman, "New Book Perpetuates Myth."

21. Carr, "The Hysterian Meets the Chronically Fatigued."

22. Kenney, K. Kimberly. "Social Security Disability: Protecting Access for PWCs." *The CFIDS Chronicle,* Summer 1996, p. 40.

23. Letters to the Editor, *New York Magazine,* August 3, 1998, p. 6.

24. Showalter, *Hystories,* p. 12.

25. Broyard, Anatole. *Intoxicated by My Illness: And Other Writings on Life and Death.* New York: Fawcett Columbine, 1992, p. 68.

26. Bly, Robert. *Leaping Poetry.* Boston: Beacon Press, 1975.

27. Lorca, Federico Garcia. *In Search of Duende.* New York: New Directions, 1998, p. 51.

28. Ibid., p. 58.

29. Hirsch, Edward. "The Duende." *American Poetry Review,* July/August 1999, p. 13.

30. Sontag, Susan. *Illness As Metaphor and AIDS and Its Metaphors.* New York: Doubleday Books, 1995, p. 3.

31. Beck, Charlotte Joko. *Nothing Special: Living Zen.* San Francisco: HarperCollins, 1993, pp. 61-71.

32. Johnson, Hillary. *Osler's Web.* New York: Crown Publishers, 1996, p. 154.

33. From the Touchtone Pictures Production Notes for *Mumford.* (Posted at Web site: <http://movieweb.com/movie/mumford/mumford.htm>.)

34. Marlette, Doug. "Kudzu." *The Washington Post,* October 17, 1997, p. E2.

35. Carlton Cards, Cleveland, Ohio. UPC# 1810084748.

36. "Hot Flashes." *OUT Magazine,* July 1999, p. 20.

37. Schmidt, Patti. "Assisted Suicide and CFIDS: Curren Death Spurs Raging Debate." *The CFIDS Chronicle,* Fall 1996, p. 9. (Comments from Mary Schweitzer.)

38. O'Neal, Allison. "Origins of Disease Names." *The CFIDS Chronicle,* Summer 1997, p. 9.

39. Bell, David S. *The Doctor's Guide to Chronic Fatigue Syndrome.* New York: Addison-Wesley Publishing, 1995, p. 7.

40. Johnson, *Osler's Web,* p. 139.

41. Ibid., p. 51.

42. Green, Judith, Jennifer Romei, and Benjamin H. Natelson. "Stigma and Chronic Fatigue Syndrome." *Journal of Chronic Fatigue Syndrome,* 5(2), 1999, pp. 63-75.

43. Johnson, *Osler's Web,* p. 135.

44. "AAFCS Conference 1998." *The CFIDS Chronicle,* January/February 1999, p. 21.

45. Hay, Louise. *You Can Heal Your Life.* Carlsbad, CA: Hay House, 1987.

46. Krakauer, Jon. *Into Thin Air.* New York: Doubleday, 1997, p. 199.

47. Burns, Roger. "Study Finds Impaired Blood Flow in CFIDS." *The CFIDS Chronicle,* Winter 1996, p. 40.

48. Norris, Chris. "Allergic to New York." *New York Magazine,* July 13, 1998, p. 33.

49. Skari, Patti. Personal communication, October 15, 1999.

50. Boxer, Sarah. "Feel Like Screaming? Excellent! You're in Demand." *The New York Times,* November 1, 1997. (From the Web site at <www.nyt.com>.)

51. Akers, Michelle. "Michelle Akers' Testimony Before Congress." (From Michelle's Web site at <www.michelleakers.com/congress.html>.)

52. Jones, Grahame L. "Achingly Good: Despite Her Battle with Chronic Fatigue, Akers Has Shown Inexhaustible Courage." *Los Angeles Times,* June 22, 1999. (From the *LA Times* Web site <www.latimes.com>.)

53. Camus, Albert. *The Plague.* Translated by Stuart Gilbert. New York: Vintage Books, 1991, p. 163.

54. Johnson, *Osler's Web,* p. 142.

55. Showalter, *Hystories,* p. 11.

56. Rotello, Gabriel. "The Birth of AIDS." *OUT Magazine,* April 1994, pp. 88-93, 130-137.

57. Callen, Michael. *Surviving AIDS.* New York: HarperCollins, 1990, pp. 5-11.

58. Ricketts, Wendell. "Living on the Edge." *OUT Magazine,* April 1994, p. 129.

59. Showalter, "Chronic Publicity Syndrome," p. 29.

60. Hoh, David. "1999 Chronicle Reader Survey." *The CFIDS Chronicle,* July/August 1999, pp. 6-9.

61. "Parkhurst Bombarded with Cures" in "Reader's Forum." *The CFIDS Chronicle,* January/February 1999, p. 3.

62. Broyard, *Intoxicated by My Illness,* p. 18.

Chapter 15

Fossil Memories

Kat Duff

Our bodies remember it all: our births, the delights and terrors of a lifetime, the journeys of our ancestors, the very evolution of life on earth. I discovered several years ago that there is a point on the inside of my knee that holds the memory and fear of a time when I was a baby and some big person lay on top of me, which I do not consciously remember. But when someone presses that point, I am suddenly there, squirming and struggling for air. Apparently I'm not the only one with trigger points for memories dotting my body like towns on a map, for gynecologist Christiane Northrup has noted that women often have memories of forgotten incest experiences during pelvic exams, explaining that procedures such as these can stir up "cellular memory, the information locked in our bodies."[1]

Our immune systems carry the memory of each and every virus we have ever encountered, and in fact every experience, from the sight of a field of daisies to the sudden shock of cold water, leaves a chemical footprint in the body, shimmering across the folds of the cortex like a wave across water, altering our attitudes, expectations, memories, and moods ever so slightly in a continual process of biological learning. Deepak Chopra, an Ayurvedic physician and MD, offered a helpful analogy to describe this process by which experiences are literally embodied: "The minutes of life (the sorrows, joys, fleeting seconds of trauma, and long hours of nothing special at all) silently accumulate and, like grains of sand deposited by a river, the minutes can eventually pile up into a hidden formation that crops above the surface"[2] as individual variations of health and illness: the straight back, wheezing cough, or fluctuating blood sugar.

Chopra also made the intriguing observation that "Memory is more permanent than matter," since formations like scars remain after all the cells that compose them are replaced, and concluded, "Your body is just the place your memory calls home."[2] This would explain how our bodies retain the memories of experience that precede our births. Recently a friend told me that when she visited the hills of Kentucky, where ancestors on both sides of her family had lived for generations, she felt an uncanny sense of familiarity, a sinking relaxation in her body, as if it remembered that landscape once called home. Another friend recalled that she developed sudden terror of heights at age forty-five, only to learn that her grandfather had watched a woman fall to her death from a building when he was that age. The body, it would seem, is a living history book.

The history encoded in our bodies is not just personal; it is also collective. Our brains contain the smaller brains of our reptilian and mammalian ancestors, what the Cherokee call our "snake and turtle minds," and we repeat their wiggling, crawling, and swinging movements in infancy, dance, and sexual play. I once looked across a room of people dancing and saw, instead, monkeys swinging from branches, otters ducking in the waves, turtles waddling across the road, and snakes slithering into rabbit holes. We also repeat these instinctual, autonomic movements in illness, when we are shivering uncontrollably, heaving over the toilet, rocking with pain, or crawling out of bed with a headache. Perhaps that is why we often speak of being reduced by illness into crybabies, slovenly beasts, or inert vegetables. Every one of us has been a tree, a fish, a deer, and much more, as the Buddhists insist, and we continue to be these things.

Sick people often speak of "crawling back through the ages" of memory, like archaeologists searching for hidden origins; as Elie Wiesel noted, "When one is ill or mad, one wants to look back as far as possible: to the brink. And beyond. Until one is back as far as possible, until one transcends the beginning."[3] When I was sickest, I lost interest in many of my usual studies, but developed a passion for reading creation myths, reveling in images of vast swirling seas of darkness, spiders spinning cosmic threads, golden eggs bursting open, a big bang at the start of time. I suspect it is no coincidence that Charles Darwin developed his theory of evolution while nearly crippled with head-aches, and the renowned physicist Stephen Hawking, who has de-voted his life to figuring out how the universe began, has an ad-vanced case of Lou Gehrig's disease. Nor is it a coincidence that the healing rituals of many traditional peoples include the retelling of creation stories.

Scientists now say that our bodies, like everything else on earth, contain atoms from the beginning of time and the origins of our universe. The elements that form our physical makeup are the same ones that constitute the earth as a living body—seawater and volcanic ash, circulating air and the spark of life that is fire—and they rank among the most powerful agents for healing, as the popularity of mineral hot springs around the world testifies. "The body is a part of the earth," explained Dr. Lewis E. Mehl, a Cherokee physician and healer. It is "the earthly home for the soul. It knows more about life on earth than the mind. When in doubt, we ask the body."[4]

My body has taught me many things, all of them filled with soul: how to dance and make love, mourn and make music; now it is teaching me how to heal. I am learning to heed the shifting currents of my body—the subtle changes in temperature, muscle tension, thought, and mood—the way a sailor rides the wind by reading the ripples on the water. Sometimes I am surprised by the feedback my body gives me; after being a vegetarian for twelve years I was astonished—and mortified—to discover that my body thrives on an occasional serving of organic red meat, at least for now. Apparently, ideology has no place in the delicate rhythms of healing.

Doctors' orders and abstract rules—such as "Get plenty of rest" or "Take daily walks"—offer helpful guidelines, but they cannot tell me when I need to change the rules; only my body can do that. That is why so many sick people come to rely upon their bodies for guidance. When Max Lerner was sick with cancer and trying to decide whether to undergo chemotherapy, he went home for a week to consult his "innermost oracle"—his body. "I recalled," he wrote, "how often I had told my seminar students to 'follow the organism.' Now I was doing that."[5]

When I was very weak and spending most of my time in bed, I used to twist and turn, stretching myself into odd positions until I found the one that was just right: curled up in a ball, arching back like a tree in high wind, or belly-up like a cat in the heat of summer. One night I dreamed that I was learning secret yoga positions reserved for the sick and dying to help them make the difficult transitions required by their stations in life; when I woke up, I realized that my body had been teaching me those poses for quite some time. This body-based learning and healing goes on all the time, but usually below the threshold of our conscious awareness; it takes an illness to draw our attention to the marvelously subtle and complex ways our bodies register changes and respond accordingly to protect the integrity of the whole.

I am often reminded that my body knows more than I do, that it has already picked up a disturbance and reacted appropriately before I realize anything is going on. For example, there have been times when I have suddenly, inexplicably, lost interest in sex, only to learn later that I am fighting an infection and need to conserve my resources, or that I am enmeshed in my relationship and need more separateness, or that I am still mad about what happened last week. Not only do our bodies know more; they also cannot lie, much to our occasional embarrassment. I have never been able to keep my voice from cracking when I am on the edge of tears, my face from flushing when a friend teases me about sex, or my hands from shaking when I am nervous. At times like that I try to remind myself: "Your body knows best. Trust it."

There are other times when it appears that my body does not know best, when I reach for that piece of chocolate cake that will make me sicker, rage at loved ones who do not deserve it, or find myself hopelessly attracted to someone I know to be cruel. Like everything that belongs to nature, our bodies have their own inexplicable streaks of madness, the uncontrollable impulses and funny quirks that save us from perfection. They are decidedly multifaceted and pluralistic, as if inhabited by many people, critters, demons, and demigods, as the ancients believed; like the ever-changing currents of water and weather, they resist our domination and persist in leading us into mystery.

NOTES

1. Christiane Northrup, "Honoring Our Bodies," *Woman of Power,* No. 18 (Fall), 1990, p. 18.

2. Deepak Chopra, *Quantum Healing* (New York: Bantom Books, 1989), p. 142.

3. Elie Wiesel, *Twilight* (New York: Warner Books, 1987), p. 213.

4. Lewis E. Mehl, "Modern Shamanism: Integration of Biomedicine with Traditional and World Views." In Gary Doore (Ed.), *Shaman's Path: Healing, Personal Growth and Empowerment* (Boston: Shambhala, 1988), p. 137.

5. Max Lerner, *Wrestling with the Angel* (New York: Simon & Schuster, 1990), p. 45.

Chapter 16

In the Shadow of Memory

Floyd Skloot

"Every day hundreds of human brains are injured," writes Howard Gardner in *The Shattered Mind*. Through accidents, strokes, tumors, or disease, people's brains, and in turn their minds and their way of experiencing the world, are altered in a flash. Nothing prepares us for this. Nothing equips us to cope with it except the very thing that has been damaged: the brain and its peculiar mesh of signals and switches that constitute our individual selves.

"The brain-damaged patient," Gardner goes on to say, "is a unique experiment in nature," allowing researchers to understand how the brain works by observing what happens when it does not. People with damaged brains offer neuroscience a deeper grasp of such human functions as language, perception, memory, mathematical or abstract reasoning, the ability to play a concerto, the ability to hit a curve ball. They expose the groundwork of "our sense of self, of the essence of our human consciousness" by revealing what happens when things "go awry."

Well, things have gone awry in me. Though I might have sought designation for uniqueness in some other way, at least I know now that my experience can be of use. Since December 1988, I have been disabled by a viral illness that targeted my brain. A nationwide research study, in which I was included as a subject, found that the brains of people with this illness were riddled with "anatomical holes" that show up as "bright lesions on magnetic resonance imaging scans of

"In the Shadow of Memory" by Floyd Skloot originally appeared in *Southwest Review,* 82(4), 1997. Reprinted with permission. Copyright Floyd Skloot, 1997.

the subcortical region." As reported to the American Society for Microbiology and in *The Journal of the American Medical Association,* researchers "do not know whether the holes will heal." Mine have not yet. A spray of holes prickles my brain and nearly everything about me has changed.

Among the functions that have been damaged, the one I am most troubled by is the corruption of memory. After more than eight years, I am still not used to it. My memory, in all its aspects, has been destabilized. My personal past, what is referred to as episodic memory, is not totally gone, but large pieces of it are. My recollection of the world I have lived in, my semantic memory, is also unreliable. Gaps exist in the historical record. Surrounding myself with reference books helps to fill them, and so does reading, but I am apt to forget what I have learned that way. Shockingly, even my ability to recall things that I have just thought or experienced, to remember faces or names or conversations or inspiration or sensation is unpredictable. I can still type without having to look at the keyboard (except for numbers) and I have managed to ride a bicycle, so my memory for tasks, my procedural memory, seems fairly well intact. Though I tend to turn a screwdriver the wrong way or to pour liquids into inverted bowls, I can perform relatively well on most activities I once performed flawlessly. But learning new tasks is monumentally difficult. From mastering the controls on our new breadmaking machine to understanding how to play Go, I am a hard study. This is not the way I used to be. Prior to 1988, I did not realize how much of my way of being in the world was predicated on a stable, functioning memory system.

In his book *The Making of Memory,* British neuroscientist Steven Rose says "memory defines who we are and shapes the way we act more closely than any other single aspect of our personhood." He adds that "we know who we are, and who other people are, in terms of memory. Lose your memory and you, as you, cease to exist." Well, it is not quite that bad for me, fortunately. I am not like some of those patients reported by Oliver Sacks, Harold Klawans, Daniel Schacter, and other students of neuroscience, patients who are fully amnesiac, lost in time or utter strangers to themselves and their families. But I am deeply altered, truly other, and this forces me to question the very integrity of my being. Now that I cannot reliably recall what happens to me, what I have set out to do or what I have actually done, or who the gentleman insisting that he is my dear childhood friend might be, who am I?

In his *Confessions,* Augustine likened memory to a great harbor receiving "in her numberless secret, and inexpressible windings all manner of sensory information, each bit entering by its own gate and laying up there for later retrieval." This notion of memory as a harbor also intrigued the great Irish painter Jack Yeats, younger brother of the poet. *Memory Harbour, 1900* is an early masterpiece collecting images that Jack Yeats would draw upon throughout his artistic career, as though the harbor itself, with its metal man on a pedestal, its captain's car and old pilot house, were a repository of one life's meaning. At a glance, the whole thing resonates for Yeats and for the viewer as well, because Yeats packs both order and emotional fullness into this cluster of remembered images from his past. "No one creates," he once said, "the artist assembles memories." This is exactly what I cannot reliably do. The harbor has been bombed. It is littered with scraps that no longer fit together.

We are on our way out to the car when I remember that I have forgotten my book bag. How am I supposed to keep a doctor's appointment without my book bag? Experience suggests that I will stay in the waiting room at least long enough to finish the novel I have been reading and begin the treatise on the nature of memory.

So I tell Beverly I forgot something, reach into my pocket for the keys while walking back toward the house, open the door, say hello to the cats, and look around the upstairs as if I had never been there before. TV is off. Lights off. Answering machine is on. Stove is cool. Though I have lived here for nearly five years, the house always astonishes me. It is round, like a double-decker wine cask made of cedar, capped with a roof that tapers to a five-foot circular skylight.

A permanent wooden yurt in the middle of twenty hilly acres of wine country, the house is technically twenty-four sided but, especially from the inside, the experience is of roundness. No sharp edges or corners, a great sense of openness and spaciousness despite its being so small. I stand in the middle of the living room looking out the south-facing wall of windows at the Eola Hills and, for the life of me, cannot recall what I am doing here. But it sure is a nice place to be. I am certain that Beverly is outside, but am I inside because was I supposed to get something? As usual, I try to reason out what is going on since I cannot recall. Already wearing my jacket, so that's not it. I check my pockets and find the vitamin holder, chock full of its many pills. Not that. Not hungry, so I wasn't after food. Must eat to keep up my health. Doctor! We are going to see the doctor. I check in my wallet to be sure I have the little red registration card that Oregon Health Science University issued to me and expects to see before I can be examined. Everything seems to be in order.

I walk back out to the car and get in. Beverly looks over at me, but does not start the engine.

"What?" I ask. The goofy, what-did-I-do-now feeling is beginning to spread down my neck like a blush.

"Where's your book bag?"

"Downstairs in the writing room. Why?"

"I thought that's what you went inside to get."

"Right." I have been through this sort of thing countless times already. So I open the car door, get the keys out while I walk, repeating over and over "book bag, book bag."

Of course, it is not just that I was distracted from remembering my book bag because we were hurrying to leave the house. We left in leisure, as we often do, anticipating a glitch. Nor was I prevented from remembering it once I had returned to the house because my mind was elsewhere; it was in some senses nowhere, or perhaps everywhere, but not truly elsewhere. Nor is this an outtake from a John Cleese routine, maybe something called *The Ministry of Feeble Brains*. I have, in recent weeks, provided myself with many other sterling examples of a short-term memory in tatters.

For example, reading the recipe for chicken cacciatore, I realized that I needed to slice a half-pound of mushrooms. By the time I turned to get them from the refrigerator, I had completely forgotten what I was after. Nothing to distract me there; the memory just slipped away like soap in the shower. A few nights ago, I thought of a brilliant idea for the start of a new essay about the way my emotions have changed since the onset of illness, and forgot the point in the few seconds it took for me to grab my pen and a chartreuse Post-it note. Maybe I should have reached for the pink ones instead. At the reception in Portland after a recent lecture by

John Updike, I shook hands with a good friend's new sweetheart, heard her name, told her I was pleased to meet her, and forgot her name before I reached the end of the sentence.

I know. It happens to everyone. But not as the norm, not predictably. If it were only a problem with short-term memory, I don't think I would mind it so much when people say, "Oh, I do that all the time." I would be able to stop myself from telling them, "Well, I didn't! Not until December 7, 1988." If it were only short-term memory that was my problem, I might not say, "Yeah, well, can you learn how to use a new camera or boom box? Can you compute change from a ten-dollar purchase? Do you lose the fifty dollars you had in your pocket while you're browsing through a bookstore? Do you forget phone numbers in the act of dialing them? Do you get lost in your own neighborhood? Do you call your cat by the name of the dog you had ten years ago?"

Numbers can be a terrible problem. I spent seventeen years (I checked; it was seventeen) working in the field of public finance and fiscal policy. At one point, I managed the budget of a $400 million state construction agency. Numbers were second nature to me until I got sick. Now I cannot get my daughter's street address right, no matter how many letters I write to her. I either transpose the numbers (131 1/2 instead of 311 1/2) or flip-flop them altogether (113 1/2 instead of 311 1/2). I can no longer add or subtract numbers in my head if they're larger than two digits, or at all if I have to "carry" numbers. We just canceled our long-distance telephone credit card and ordered a new one; if I use if often enough, I may have its fourteen numbers memorized by the time the new millennium begins. With my agent's telephone number on a card before me, I added it to my speed dialing system incorrectly and ended up calling a New York City garbage collection company, which was perhaps more of a symbolic error than I would care to admit. The proper term for my selective difficulty in dealing with numbers is "acalculia." But I prefer to believe that I multiply and divide numbers the way a new Chinese immigrant speaks English, as if I'd never really seen the alphabet before, as if I couldn't quite form the sounds. So I think of my math as having an accent.

Learning new tasks is often beyond my capabilities. We do not tend to realize that such learning is a function of memory, but it is—procedural memory, they call it, or skill memory. So not only is my memory for *naming* unreliable, my memory for *doing* is compromised as well. When I bought a more sophisticated computer last year, the process of learning how to use it nearly drove me nuts and I still cannot use WordPerfect 6.0 efficiently, relying on the 5.1 that I knew before getting sick. Weeks of repetition were needed for me to learn how to use my new fax capabilities, though the process requires all of four simple steps. Same with Beverly's VCR, despite four years of trying, since it operates differently from my own. Use it, hell, I am incapable of calling up the menu properly. I cannot light and manage the fire in our woodstove, though Beverly has repeatedly shown me how to do it, and though I once wrote the steps down on an index card (which I have lost). My failures to learn simple tasks frustrate me and make me feel as if I am letting her down, no matter how often she tells me otherwise.

I forget which people I have told what item of news, repeating myself shamelessly. I forget to do anything that I have not written down in my calendar book, on the Post-it notes that festoon my living spaces, in the notebooks I keep on the bedside table or on the living room credenza or on the washing machine, in the bathroom, or in the glove compartment of the car. For weeks, a friend was telling me about her forthcoming book tour to Seattle and Bellingham, yet when she hadn't sent me any e-mail for five straight days I became very concerned, completely forgetting that she was gone. I forget what day or month it is. I forget my dreams. Follow directions? Give me a break.

It is the summer of 1988, a warm July evening, and I have just turned forty-one years old. Within the last year, I have run my fastest marathon, and my fastest ten-, eight- and five-kilometer races ever, winning ribbons for my age group in the latter three categories. I am on a roll. Lining up with other "masters runners" on the track at Lincoln High School, I am about to run a mile race for the first time in my life. Uncertain how to do it, how to pace myself since I'm used to the longer distances, I decide to shoot for a conservative time of 5:20 and to run each lap at an identical pace of 1:20 per lap.

When the gun sounds, I take off and set my internal clock, falling into a stride that feels right for the goal. Halfway around the first lap, I glance at my watch: thirty-two seconds. In my head, I calculate quickly: slow down just a bit, and finish the lap exactly as the official calls out eighty seconds. Bingo. To keep myself occupied and distracted, I begin to calculate what my times would be if I could sustain a 5:20 pace for a five kilometer-race, converting miles to meters in my head, dividing accurately, multiplying accurately while I run and listen to the times being called and even hear distinctly the cheers from my friends who have come to support me. Holding steady, I finish the race in 5:19, take my pulse as I walk around the track, and calculate how long it should take to return to resting count.

Exactly six months later, to the day, I got sick in a hotel room in Washington, DC. I was fine on the long flight from Portland, fine during the evening as I prepared for a conference on national energy policy. But I woke up transformed. It was 6:00, and I knew I should go out for a brisk five-mile run around the mall, but I could not remember how to shut off the alarm on my wrist watch, beeping at me ominously from the bedside table. Too exhausted to fold back the covers, I tried to determine what time it was back home in Oregon, see if that explained why I felt so tired, but could not figure it out. Was 6:00 here, so it was . . . I could remember neither whether to add or subtract, nor how much, nor what the alternative sums or remainders might be. I finally got up, put on my running gear, and sat on the edge of the bed trying to understand how to make my shoes stay on, since tying the laces was proving impossible. I tried to put my blue wristband over my head like a headband and could not understand how it had shrunk so much on the flight across country. I tried to open the room door by pressing on its hinges; I tried to get on the elevator before the doors parted.

At work the next week, I could barely perform simple tasks. Familiar phone numbers—for the lobbyists in seven states with whom I regularly consulted, the vice president of government affairs to whom I reported, my grown son in his new apartment—were forgotten. I erased a brief memo on my computer, a memo I could not finish anyway but wanted to save in order to develop later, when I felt better. I got lost walking the few blocks down toward the shop where I always went to have coffee. In a meeting to discuss proposed changes to federal regulations on electric power, I was unable to grasp the basic concepts being discussed—power pricing policy, power sales—concepts with which I had been dealing for three years. At the snack bar on the mezzanine, I could not remember how to choose the bag of pretzels I came to buy, nor figure out how to work the machine.

Within six weeks, I had performed so poorly on a neuropsychological exam that the administering doctor, Muriel Lezak, the highly respected author of a 1983 Oxford University Press textbook, *Neuropsychological Assessment,* explained my results with real astonishment. It was, she felt, a strange assortment of "significant cognitive problems" and an abnormal "difficulty in keeping track of ongoing mental activity." What she called my "severe visual learning disability," and "great difficulty in organizing and synthesizing visual material when the burden of making structure is on him," I experienced as virtually total alienation from the person I knew myself to be. Nothing made sense anymore. I was lost in time and space, it seemed; I felt myself, my mind, to be incoherent and my world to be in fragments.

"Remember," Dr. Lezak said, looking at me across her desk, her dark, tired eyes suddenly softening, "inefficiency in mental processing is not stupidity."

Always a person drawn to order and structure, a poet whose work often rhymed and had traditional formal organization, a novelist given to carefully constructed narratives, I would have to learn to yield to the fragmentation of my experience, viewing it as a kind of antiorder. Randomness, elusiveness, and impermanence announced themselves as essential truths; my quest would have to be for understanding, not order.

One of the strangest aspects of living with certain kinds of memory loss is knowing that the forgetting is happening. I know I am not going to remember things that I desperately want to remember and have only limited success in using special encoding techniques to hold on to what matters. Memories of the last visits with my brother in San Jose, for instance, where he is dying from complications of diabetes. We visit him every three months as his condition worsens—he is now on dialysis four days a week, blind, nearly immobile, not always alert—and each visit feels like it could be the last. We sit together in his living room and talk, but by the time I return to my room and take notes it is too late. I long to hoard what we say, how he looks, the things we are able finally to communicate. But no matter how hard I try to focus, to encode and keep safe these memories that are so packed with meaning for me, the results are mixed at best, and what remains is usually what Beverly recalls for me.

I find myself highlighting nearly the entire text of a book in yellow, repeating to myself each idea there, closing my eyes and saying it over and over, yet an hour later, when I pick up the book again, I have little recall of what the point was. Something about patients who deny the existence of deficits, a woman lying in bed with a paralyzed left side but insisting that the only reason she could not move her left arm was that it was tired today. I realize it is wondrously ironic to forget details of a chapter on amnesia, but at the time the humor escaped me.

In addition, I know I am making mistakes and cannot prevent them. This morning, I told Beverly that I would take out the baggage instead of the garbage, but by now she is so used to my malapropisms that she did not seem to notice. Last month, crossing a street at the designated area, leading with my cane, I assured her that the rapidly oncoming cars would stop for us since we were in the car wash. Of course I meant to say crosswalk; I heard myself goof and grimly corrected myself, but this sort of thing is now common with me. I have called the refrigerator a storm drain; called a concerto a rintoletto, which sounds like a wonderful thing but does not even exist; and—a catastrophic mistake for me—called the Brooklyn Dodgers the Boxers. When I announced that *the carbon came dewy,* I meant to say that *the barbecue had gotten moldy* over the winter, while we had it stored in the shed. These "paraphasias" of mine, these substitutions of a word or creations of new words related in sound and meaning to the intended word, concern me when I am speaking in front of an audience, especially when I read from my own work. I feel only minimally in control of my word-finding capacities, or my ability to remember words and concepts. I am safe with them only when I am alone and writing, able to correct myself before anyone sees or hears the mistakes.

My penchant for such gobbledygook is hardly confined to words. I make similar mistakes with directions while traveling by car, certain that we must turn right when it is not only the wrong direction for where we are going, but a one-way street as well. It's a kind of spatial paraphasia, I suppose, a confusion that is not corrected by traveling familiar roads. No matter how many times we drive to visit Beverly's parents, I cannot find my way around the lake on which they live. I will emerge from a grocery store parking lot and feel certain that the highway is behind us, though I can see and hear the traffic ahead. I sometimes find myself throwing together an odd gestural salad, my hand movements wrong for what I am saying, like an orchestra conductor performing a golf swing when he wants the woodwinds to join in.

Memory is required in order to think in the way we are accustomed to think. The sum of my experiences, the store of knowledge I have accumulated, the training and discipline of thought that have shaped the kind of person or the kind of writer I became—all these require an access to memory that is no longer routine for me. You cannot think if you cannot remember; at best, you can react.

I find myself unable to work my way through certain problems, especially those requiring abstract thought. A psychiatrist hired by the Social Security Administration to reevaluate my disability status last year asked me to explain what is meant by the expression "people who live in glass houses shouldn't throw stones." Well, hell, I know what that means! Metaphor is my game. But I could not actually explain how the concept worked, why the metaphor was apt, or what the proverb meant. It was as though my interpretive faculties had vanished. I could not think. I could not find words to describe what I saw, or remember how to approach the problem and begin to reason it out. I fumbled around for five minutes before he finally spared me further embarrassment and frustration.

When Beverly and I watch movies, I am a textbook example of memory's malfunctions. Though a passionate student of film, I have trouble naming movies in which I've seen an actor whose work I admire and hardly ever can recall an individual director's previous work. This is a topic in which I was well versed before getting sick. I lose the thread of narrative; foreshadowing is wasted on me. Sometimes, Beverly will miss a scrap of dialogue and ask me what was said; I can repeat back flawlessly several sentences at a time, provided she asks me within about five seconds of hearing the speech. But I cannot remember a word of it, despite having already said the speech myself, about ten or twenty seconds later. We tried an experiment, once this occurred to me, and shut off the sound after I repeated a speech, so that there would be little distraction. Gone in twenty seconds. This is a fine example of an intact "working memory"—that storehouse of transient information in memory's busy harbor which is quickly raided for material that will be stored, or encoded into the short-term or long-term memory banks—working with a damaged encoding system. These are functions controlled by different parts of the brain. So I can often retain material for a few seconds, but fail to organize and categorize the information correctly and therefore lose it. If there are any distractions—music playing, other people talking nearby, movement outside the window, a gesture of the hand, a competing thought—I will almost certainly lose what I might otherwise remember. This is no significant loss when all that is at stake is a few lines of dialogue from a movie. But the same thing happens when I read, for example, and have great difficulty retaining new information, losing the thread of plot or character, failing to absorb important data, key facts (the hippocampus is where?). It also happens when I converse with someone, when I get a flash of inspiration that should be retained, an idea for something I want to write, a line of poetry.

These are unnerving occurrences, regardless of their frequency. I know that I knew what I no longer know. It is there as a kind of shadow memory, something at the edges of awareness, elusive and troubling. Many of my memories seem to be like this, whether immediate or short-term or long-term; memory is often a vague, partly hidden, distorted realm for me. And threatening at times, because I never can be sure when it will function well. I have had to learn how to be in public again, how to shed the shame and anxiety that memory loss engenders and work with what I have available.

What all this suggests, and what I have learned intimately, is that human memory is not one thing but many things, a system, a layered or modular set of functions. We may experience memory as a fluid and continuous thing, a film or an album or a script, but it is in fact a delicately wired arrangement of separate operations. To experience it as such is terribly strange. As Daniel L. Schacter explains in his brilliant book *Searching for Memory,* "we have now come to believe that memory is not a single or unitary faculty, as was long assumed. Instead, it is composed of a variety of distinct and dissociable processes and systems. Each system depends on a particular constellation of networks in the brain that involve different neural structures, each of which plays a highly specialized role within the system." But that is not how it feels to most of us, until things go wrong, until there are things like holes in the brain that interrupt the flow.

For me, the damage seems to be almost everywhere, but not too deep. All sorts of system components seem slightly off, but no one component has broken down fully. I do not think it is always 1956, or fail to recognize faces while readily recognizing voices; I do not mistake my wife for a hat. But I have a little of all these people in me, as though my brain had been scattershot, messing up the connections but not utterly destroying anything.

You lose an old photograph of yourself at four, perched on a tricycle with your father, who would die in the next few years, crouched beside you and smiling at the camera. You break the gravy boat inherited from your grandmother, the maroon Myott/Staffordshire with gold trim in a bouquet pattern that you remember seeing drip on her linen tablecloth in the apartment on Central Park West. You lose the scent or feel of a lover's presence, an old friend's voice, the precise contours of your sister's face. When this happens, it feels as though you have lost a bit of yourself, so fragile is the material of memory.

In early 1990, I received a letter from the owner of a major Manhattan art gallery. He had seen three of my poems and an essay in recent issues of *The New Criterion* and wondered if I was the Floyd Skloot who grew up in Long Beach, New York. Because if so, then I was his best friend. His name, Larry Salander, sounded vaguely familiar, but I could not remember anything more about him. I called my mother, who, at eighty, not only remembered Larry but remembered his father as well because Mr. Salander had bought all our furniture when we were forced to move after my father's death. She told me that I had played on a basketball team with Larry and sent along a clipping about us that she had saved since 1964.

I wrote to Larry, saying that I was the Floyd Skloot from Long Beach (How could there be another person with such a name, after all?), but that I had no memory of him. Certainly, I could have written more tactfully, or more fully, but I was bedridden at the time. He says that he threw my letter in the wastebasket and was deeply offended, furious that I did not remember him. But then he calmed down and wrote back anyway to explain that he had been my neighbor, my playmate and teammate. He recalled being in my house with me the evening after my father died. He was filled with the memories I had lost and, when I explained my situation, was eager to share them. In the seven years that followed, Larry not only helped me reclaim many of those memories, he resumed his place in my life as a friend so close that I cannot get through a week without talking to him. His own paintings have graced the covers of my last two books. In many ways, Larry is a symbol for me of all that can be lost, of the preciousness and tenuousness of memory, but also of hope, since he is back and so is some of what I had lost.

As I turn fifty, the world and my place in it look much different than I had imagined they would. I have come to place tremendous value on the intensity and power of the moment, since I can never be sure a moment will last in memory. It must be savored now and to do that I have had to simplify my life, slow it down and reduce the number of things competing for attention. The more complex my life becomes, the more of it eludes me. I live in the country now, in rural isolation two miles outside a town of 1,100 people, with no neighbors closer than a quarter mile. My old calendar books, the kind with one week spread across each page to allow for all the entries, has been replaced by a thin monthly calendar book with tiny boxes for each day. Blank boxes far outnumber filled ones.

I try to resist the feeling that, in losing so many elements of memory's function, I have lost myself, that I am adrift. Without Beverly's abiding love and support, I am sure it would be much more difficult to feel anchored. But at times the sense of having a scrambled memory, of its unpredictable and unreliable performance, makes me feel eroded. Or perhaps the more accurate word is haunted. In his book *Memory's Ghost*, Philip J. Hilts studies examples of memory loss and comments on the "haunting moments, and haunted lives" he has witnessed. Quoting the early French student of memory, Dr. Theodule Ribot, Hilts describes "how memory loss can pierce our sense of solidity, can invade our belief that we are who we are, that all goes on as before." Memory loss moves through everything else like a ghost; nothing can stop it. It insinuates itself into life moment by moment, invisible to others except in how it makes its host respond. Having lost the integrity of my mental process, my past and often my present, I sometimes sense images floating away like ghosts too, the familiar transformed in a flash to the strange. I am haunted by what I have missed, though it happened to me.

Oliver Sacks refers to a patient suffering from an extraordinary loss of recent memory as having lost "his moorings in time." He also says that "to be ourselves we must *have* ourselves—possess, if need be, repossess, our life-stories. We must 'recollect' ourselves, recollect the inner drama, the narrative, of ourselves." This is what we need to hold on to, by hook or by crook, if we are to keep whole. People with memories damaged by injury or illness usually tell their stories only to their physicians, loved ones, or friends. By telling it more widely, I am not only helping myself remember, I am bearing witness, and trying to reclaim my humanity, bringing it out of the shadows of lost memories and into the light of experience.

PART IV:
SYNERGY AND MOVEMENT

Chapter 17

On Life, Death, and the Nature of Limbo: Assisted Suicides in the CFIDS Community

Peggy Munson

Even serious Internet stories read like a transcribed game of telephone, so when I heard about Bill's death, I refused to believe it.

I knew Bill by his online moniker but not by his real name, and even though I didn't *know* him, I doubted he would turn to the famous suicide doctor to stop his pain. He was, by my estimation, a lot like me. "BostonBill" and I were members of the same self-appointed oligarchy of support group leaders on America Online. My own group had been running two years, so I shared e-mail ephemera and goodwill with the other fibromyalgia, multiple chemical sensitivity, and chronic fatigue immune dysfunction syndrome (CFIDS) chat leaders. Bill was a proactive organizer with severe fibromyalgia who experienced unrelenting pain. I convinced myself that the news reports, which named him as Dr. Jack Kevorkian's latest assisted suicide, were just medical tall tales, like the Internet Invasion of the Kidney Snatchers stories that had recently entered cyber legend. BostonBill was lost before I ever got to know his real name, his quirks, or what his family thought of his decision to die.

People with chronic illness live in a state of limbo. We are like residents of a dense fog. We can be remarkably close without seeing each other, without being seen, and danger may be ominously proximate, or not near at all. We do not know what lies in front of us and our lives are gauzy and uncertain. It is easier to crash into us than to perceive our true parameters. We are denied the stages of common heroism that healthy people experience during the flu—the temporary altered consciousness, the bad temper, the hard-core vitamin consumption, the wonderful existential musings, and the inevitable triumph of immunity. Things do not shift back for us. Our homeostasis goes haywire. We may be indefinitely suspended in a world of political torture. But our foreign country, the one that holds us hostage and begs our secrets and private dignity, is the body we once trusted, now possessed by a strange, turncoat dictator.

Because of this limbo, communication among online sick and disabled people resembles that of trucker culture—sometimes hours are spent connecting with strangers over the wire, snatching bits and pieces of community culture from the strange, encapsulate reality that permeates homebound living. Before I contracted CFIDS, I dismissed the notion of cybercommunity as a myth of the technological age. In college, I studied intentional community building by reading about nineteenth-century utopian societies, living briefly on a remote commune, and cooking vast quantities of tofu for a college co-op. This all changed abruptly when my dizzy spells before graduation evolved into a full-fledged debilitating horror. As I became increasingly homebound and finally plugged into the online revolution, I learned that "real" community can happen electronically. While I sometimes longed for the type of rural society in which my parents grew up, where church groups would visit the sick with casseroles and prayers, I found myself living alone, quite debilitated, and a thousand miles from that familiar homeland. The cybercommunity I helped to create became, for me, a saving grace.

BostonBill and I had exchanged a few personal notes. His last one urged me to forward a new pain treatment protocol to as many people as I could. So, while we were not friends in real time, he was a living member of the main community I had. And furthermore, he was the first person with whom I had made personal contact in this community to commit suicide.

The *CFIDS Chronicle* ran a postcard-sized story about Boston-Bill soon after his death. There, I learned his real name was Bill Connaughton, he resided in West Roxbury, Massachusetts, and he was only forty-two years old. *The Chronicle* reported that Bill was "known for the support, cheerfulness and advice he offered through online chat rooms he had organized for people with fibromyalgia."[1]

Because of his excruciating pain, Bill believed his body was riddled with tumors, though an autopsy showed no sign of tumorous growths. Nevertheless, even dosages of painkillers described as "potentially lethal" could not temper his fibromyalgia. Dr. Kevorkian, the notorious and controversial Dr. Death, provided a final and irreversible analgesic.

The kind of pain people experience with CFIDS and fibromyalgia is often inexplicable. In the online chat rooms, many of us feel like children whining, "it hurts," but don't know how to convey how, or why. It's very hard to translate, and it's often the kind of pain that's so bad you just can't talk about it. I know a lot of fiercely tough people online who would shatter any myths about CFIDS being a ragdoll malady, but they are too sick, too brain-fogged, and too beaten down to defend their own experiences. Most of us have agonized over the suicides in the CFIDS community. There have been far too many of them—most unpublicized because they didn't involve Kevorkian. Numerous CFIDS sufferers sit at home with the tools, the pills, and an explicit internal methodology. Suicides are often a shrill and powerful voice of mobility, a chance to be a revolutionary martyr when one can barely get out of bed. In this way, they can be highly seductive to the homebound. As Anne Sexton put it, "Suicides have a special language./Like carpenters they want to know *which tools*./They never ask *why build*."[2]

Connaughton was the third in a trinity of Kevorkian-assisted suicides in my illness community. In August 1996, Kevorkian made headlines with the assist of Judith Curren, a disabled forty-two-year-old registered nurse from Pembroke, Massachusetts, who suffered from CFIDS and fibromyalgia. Because the coroner wrongly stated that Curren was "not ill" and her condition was not considered terminal, even Kevorkian supporters believed he had finally crossed a sacred line. Although Curren quite possibly enlisted Dr. Death's help to get national attention for the pain of CFIDS sufferers, her strategy backfired. CFIDS became a target of national ridicule, as it had so many times before, when newspapers disparaged the legitimacy of her diagnoses and Rush Limbaugh said that everyone he knew with CFIDS "was fat and lazy before they got sick."[3]

Curren's death was also clouded by reports that she may have been a victim of domestic assault, though her husband pronounced that their spousal fights had been motivated by his disapproval of her desire to seek Kevorkian's help. Several doctors at the 1998 American Association of Chronic Fatigue Syndrome (AACFS) conference did report that domestic violence is a real concern for people with CFIDS.[4] Abuse may be triggered by a spouse's frustration toward a disabled partner who looks perfectly healthy. Perhaps this behavior mimics that of predatorial animals, who target lame prey first. In reports of Curren's death, though, the abuse allegations simply muddied the story, and they were never confirmed. Her husband's statements were highly plausible, and it was hard to say whether or not he, too, was a victim of the media circus. Papers launched a tabloid parody of Judith's life.

Less than a year later, a Nevada woman with CFIDS and fibromyalgia was found dead with a note on her chest instructing authorities to call Kevorkian's lawyer. Dr. Death's involvement in her suicide was not confirmed, but Janis Murphy, age forty, was believed to be the second Kevorkian-assisted CFIDS suicide.[5] When I received word of her death over the Internet, I delayed forwarding it to my eighty-some list members. Curren's death had sparked other, less publicized, suicides in the CFIDS community, and I feared Murphy's death would do the same. I was particularly worried about one group member who frequently came to the chat room with loud and vibrant suicidal ideations. Like the magical realist world of Gabriel García Márquez's *One Hundred Years of Solitude,* where insomnia becomes a contagious illness, I knew that in the surreal, purgatorial world of the chronically ill, suicide was contagious too. I didn't want to pass on its virulent pathogen.

Murphy's death happened almost exactly ten months after Curren's, and Bill Connaughton's death happened about ten months after Murphy's. Ten became a numerological death card. As time passed, I began to despair that the pendulum would swing again, and I barely skimmed new *Chronicles,* quit my group leadership, and delved heavily into weekly psychotherapy to deal with my own illness grief. Around that time, I reconnected with a friend who had been sick even longer than I had. Like everyone else I knew, she took a hard line on Kevorkian, calling him a *murderer.* Though I agreed Kevorkian's zeal reflected a perverse megalomania, I secretly wondered if he was doing some people with CFIDS a favor. Sometimes, I fantasized about ending the seven-year horror of my battle with this disabling, invisible illness. And sometimes, lying still for hours near the phone thinking I might be dying anyway, I barely found the strength to scribble out notes to my friends and family telling them that if I died of uncertain causes, to know that it wasn't a suicide. I knew I wouldn't choose suicide and I really wanted to *live*. But I often felt so sick I believed I must be dying. My real fear was that I would die before I had the chance to ride my bike again.

People understand why a prisoner would choose suicide, but critics are very hard on the chronically ill. It's hard to comprehend the way illness robs one of simple freedoms. Sure, society understands visible shackles—they get the symbolism of the wheelchair, of prosthetics, of a bumper sticker reading *disabled veteran,* but they still struggle for comprehension of the profound, invisible shackles that an illness such as CFIDS puts on a person's body. This is part of the nature of living in limbo. Once, when I took a class about fear of flying, an instructor explained to me how wind is an actual *substance,* and clouds weigh as much as large buildings. But try to explain the weight of clouds to a skeptic moving his hand through the steam of his daily, hard-earned coffee, and you will have an inkling of the kind of justifications CFIDS patients are forced to make. Then try explaining this when you have flu symptoms, severe cognitive problems, the exhaustion of someone who just ran the Boston marathon, and the stamina of a severe cardiac patient, and you will know why CFIDS patients may appear unduly frustrated. For people with CFIDS, there is no Dr. Life, only Dr. Death, and this is the fundamental quandary. The only doctor supplying real relief from the grueling pain is the one who ends it permanently. People with CFIDS need more options.

In America, we ignore the invisible things that hinder independence, clinging to the great myth that independence is viable for anyone with enough will. Viewed as speed treads along the parkway of the American Dream, people with disabilities are thus told they should strive for "independent living." For those with CFIDS, who are covered under the Americans with Disabilities Act (ADA) but for whom garnering support services and disability benefits is a disheartening battle, independence is often a rhetorical abstraction. No Alcatraz is as inescapable as one's own debilitated body.

But there were other reasons why Bill Connaughton's death got under my skin. I had lost another Bill who, like Connaughton, feared the unknown and suspected a terminal condition that didn't exist. He had an improbable ten-letter surname. Bill's was eleven letters. I could not help but notice that ten, that death card, was the number at the high threshold of pain scales, signaling a level of distress that was intolerable.

I grew up in the geographical center of the American Dream, where the land was squared off, scraped with thick metal tines, fecund and magical. McLean County, Illinois, with some of the richest farmland in the country, was expansive. Fourteen years ago in that piece of the heartland, as summer reached its humid peak, my life changed irrevocably. Since Independence Day, I'd been finding empty firecracker shells near the creek bridge by my house. That summer was hot and itchy, dense with meteorological fore-shadowing, as if the weather was tuned in to the devious youthful energy that crept up in the silence after school bells. Everybody had secret plans then, but nobody talked about them; we didn't want to risk being struck down. Some of us were impudent dreamers. At night, in the impossibly flat darkness, in the center of the nation which felt like nowhere, we could always see a little bit too far for our own good.

About a week after Independence Day, in a trailer court across town, my grandfather pulled out a gun, walked into the bathroom, and shot himself. I woke to my sister Molly's cries in the bedroom adjoining mine. Molly had just received Grandma's hysterical reve-lation that her husband—our grandfather—was dead on the bath-room floor. With hospice diplomacy and quiet faith, Molly often seemed to field the emergency calls in my house.

Other members of my family possessed a macabre parapsychology. In fact, my grandmother and I had both had premonitions of my grandfather's death. That May or June, I dreamed he was careening through space and woke up fearing his death. My grandmother, who was out late playing cards the night he took his life, remembers sitting down very suddenly in a chair, as if the wind had been knocked out of her, around the time the gun went off. She didn't find his body until the next morning. A resilient survivor who emanated quiet respectability, my grandmother would never disparage the value of a good night's sleep.

The day was heavy with the kind of atmospheric density that happens before summer storms rip across the plains. My grandfather had been a tenant farmer on the vast prairie for years, a quiet and giving man who spoke rarely but purposefully. His actions tended to be direct and guided, and his life was rhythmic and ritualistic, like that of most agrarians. On his suicide day, we emulated his directive Protestantism and went to work. My mother drove over to the trailer to console her mother and deal with the authorities. My sister and I, who were both still in high school, helped out at my mother's retail store, quietly unpacking boxes and stocking food on the shelves.

I don't remember crying much that day. I also don't remember being told the death was a suicide, though I later found out. Soon after his death, I stealthily went to the library to xerox an article the local paper ran about him, an article I had chanced upon that morning at breakfast, scanning it quickly and folding the paper shut. The coroner's office, apparently without my family's permission, released his suicide note, which the paper printed in its entirety. In the short note, my grandfather spoke of his fear of being a burden to his family. A seventy-two-year-old man of reasonably good health, he had spent several weeks in a high-tech Chicago hospital a few years before to have surgery on his heart. I remember listening to the monitors beep around his pale body and thinking how out of place he looked in that urban hospital, like a prospector in a time warp.

He said he was afraid he might have cancer because of blood in his urine, or that the artificial valve in his heart was failing. Terrified of becoming a burden to the family, not wanting to be stuck in a nursing home, he decided to take matters into his own hands. My grandfather was not one to cry wolf. He didn't give any of us a chance to talk him out of it. His suicide was sudden, inexplicable, and irreversible. The man who had represented the essential rigidity of bygone days had acted unpredictably for the first time and last time, as far as I can remember, that I ever witnessed. I will never get over it.

Patience is the hardest part of having a chronic condition. Despite the axioms I was raised on, such as "virtue is its own reward," I could find little virtue in the suffering of my illness, and certainly no reward. When I first became ill, I absorbed a lot of the cultural backlash against the illness, and tried to convince myself I was "just depressed." I had been depressed before; my family tree sagged beneath an ice storm of clinical depression. One of Grandpa's siblings also committed suicide; another was institutionalized. A cousin of mine went through bouts of severe depression. The connections between these events were never discussed in my family. Denial is perhaps the most popular antidote against mental illness, and we practiced, like a quilting circle in after hours, simply hemming everything in.

People in the CFIDS community are afraid of talking publicly about depression. Because early government reports dismissed us as psychosomatic and mentally ill, it is hard to admit being depressed without being publicly discredited, even though numerous scientists have outlined the clinical differences between CFIDS and primary depression. Almost anybody would experience depression with the level of grief and loss CFIDS people deal with. Most of us lose our jobs, some of our friends, the capacity to enjoy simple activities, and a great degree of our freedom to act spontaneously. Many lose the support of primary partners. Many lose financial security, fighting for years to get disability benefits, which generally only amount to subpoverty wages. Some end up homeless. These circumstances make some grief and depression almost inevitable. Researchers postulate that CFIDS affects brain chemistry as well. How this brain dysfunction tampers with mood is still poorly conceptualized.

Despite popular mythology, though, CFIDS is *not* a form of depression. It is a separate entity altogether. Most people with CFIDS do not have a history of depression, or a family history of depression. My case was unusual. But because of my own background, I was already bilingual in the "special language" of suicides. As an online CFIDS support group leader, I was torn apart whenever I heard the desperate voice of someone with CFIDS considering death. As a suicide survivor, it pulled at my most complicated emotions. As a person with CFIDS, I was unsure what to say to talk the person out of it. I couldn't necessarily guarantee the person would feel differently in a week or a month. I could only offer my own metaphor about CFIDS being like catastrophic weather. It comes in like a tornado; it could leave just as quickly.

Strict clinical differences distinguish CFIDS from depression, such as specific profiles on psychological, immunological, and neurological tests, or the fact that people with depression tend to respond positively to exercise, which often exacerbates CFIDS symptoms and causes decreased blood flow to the patients' brains. CFIDS patients generally *want* to do things, but are too sick, whereas people with primary depression tend to lose the desire to participate in activities. CFIDS patients have ongoing flulike symptoms such as sore throats, severe headaches, chronic pain, nausea, and irritable bowel-type symptoms, uncommon to those with primary depression. In addition, CFIDS patients exhibit measurable brain impairment such as slowed information processing, abstract reasoning problems, loss of IQ points, and difficulty using words and numbers, indicating that "the inner workings of the brain are weak."[6] Still, with any illness, the prospect of *secondary* depression is foreboding. With an illness as maligned and untreatable and disabling as CFIDS, secondary depression is a frequent phenomenon and needs to be treated as the serious and potentially life-threatening condition that it is.[7]

Although psychiatry may play a role in helping people with CFIDS cope with their losses, society has become so preoccupied with denigrating CFIDS that they have followed a historical precedent of shuffling misunderstood conditions into the psychiatric field. Dr. Alan Gurwitt, a child psychiatrist, queried, "Why this morbid, tiresome and destructive preoccupation with ferreting out any shred of evidence of psychiatric difficulties? Would not the all too limited [CFIDS] research funds better be devoted to furthering biological research already in progress or waiting to be funded, or devoted to developing ways to improve physician interest and education?"[8]

I think people with CFIDS also need to look at the bigger picture. As Jan Montgomery, a CFIDS activist, stated, "If normal people get a flat tire, they call AAA. If CFIDS patients get a flat tire, they call suicide prevention."[9] Although people with CFIDS certainly need better medical options, they also need to consider that cultivating patience may be a key to survival and recovery. There certainly is hope for us, but we might have to wait.

I do not blame my grandfather, though I have gone through anger, disbelief, rage, fear, and grief. These are similar to the feelings that raged through the CFIDS community following each of Kevorkian's assisted suicides. I wonder what would have happened if my grandfather had hung on for a few more years, until the media paid more attention to depression. The man who used to sit beside the television set and listen to it like an old radio died several years before *Listening to Prozac* hit the best-seller list. Because of this, I cannot help wondering which medication, held up in the rusty cogs of beaurocracy, might have saved Connaughton, or Curren, or Murphy if they had waited a little bit longer.

Although I recognize the inherent danger in comparing Bill Connaughton's suicide to my grandfather's, I think both have something to say about limbo. People who live in limbo both court and fear death, because they are forced to live in the same house with it, and it is a troubling cohabitant. One Buddhist monk was said to have meditated while lying on the dead body of his mother, over a period of days, to come to terms with the reality of death. Few people experience this kind of reckoning with physical decay. CFIDS is an ongoing meditation on the body's unknowns, and it has a lot to teach the healthy population. It remains one of the most misunderstood and elusive illnesses of our time. It also remains one of the most hated. When I read the notes of other CFIDS suicide victims, printed in the *CFIDS Chronicle,* I could not help but notice that the victims had chosen a demonstrative tragedy to represent the living tragedy of CFIDS. They went to such lengths not only to find relief, but to convince the public of the tragedy that CFIDS was for them. Nobody should be forced to turn to such measures. People with CFIDS should be offered treatments, fair disability payments, and most of all, recognition and dignity.

Even the Social Security Administration has a hard time understanding limbo. When I applied for benefits, after struggling for three years to work part-time despite grueling symptoms, they kept insisting that I could lift boxes, stand on my feet for hours, and work an eight-hour day, even though I was unable to do any of those things. When I applied for benefits, I had in fact been offered a partial fellowship at Columbia University's graduate School of the Arts, and would have given anything to not concede defeat and to continue my education instead. My lawyer told me that if I had lost a leg, and been a waitress, I would have sailed right through the process, as the SSA would just plug me into a simple equation and offer benefits. As it was, they were facing my strange limbo, and they kept turning me down. My lawyer told me, when we went into the hearing with an administrative law judge, that they would likely try to assert that I could assemble boxes at home to earn a viable income.

"They will want me to be a box maker?" I said, aghast.

"I've seen it happen before," said my lawyer.

Luckily, I never became a box maker, but the sad fact is that I couldn't have even done it if I wanted to. I was too *sick* to assemble boxes at home. My doctor wrote on one form, "must rest continuously." This state of rest—the body in rest, and not in motion—characterizes the viral purgatory of CFIDS. Sometimes I think we may as well be box makers. Our efforts appear empty to the outside world. Our cheeks, our visage, our voices all seem hollow until the public looks closer. To the unknowing eye, we are goods in transit, because we are neither healthy nor dead. We are just something packed up in the 1980s and shoved into a corner, perhaps the disheveled postsurgical photographs of an otherwise healthy person. We represent the part of life most healthy people would like to forget.

Unfortunately, the silence and invisibility of CFIDS patients has effectively been perceived as tacit agreement with the status quo. People may interpret CFIDS suicides to mean that CFIDS victims will just quietly disappear, that they are "just depressed" and somewhat of a social embarrassment. In this respect, these skeletons have locked their own closet doors. People with CFIDS who kill themselves are the millennium's favorite type of disabled citizens—those who will walk quietly among the healthy, then quietly dispose of themselves. However, this makes survivors with CFIDS particularly irritating to the social norm when they act up and make noise, and especially when they express disbelief and depression. In a Darwinistic world, which is largely predatorial, the only thing worse than an invisible game animal is one who stirs the hunter's conscience.

I think it is time we stirred the hunter's conscience and furthermore, brought him into our fog. But vampire legends aside, it is hard for the undead to inflict the living, and few of us would want that. And I am only half-joking when I refer to us as the undead. Dr. David Bell, one of the most noted CFIDS researchers, has found a large percentage of CFIDS patients to have extremely low blood volume, perhaps even less than a person who has nearly bled to death.[10] But as long as CFIDS is perceived as a Raggedy Ann disease, bad boys will pull at the doll's yarn hair and pound her stuffed flesh. It is no wonder that CFIDS, seen as the ragdoll malady, was quickly placed among pop psychological constructions such as Peter Pan syndrome. CFIDS must be seen simply for what it is: a devastating physical illness that can make the most mentally stable people contemplate suicide. CFIDS patients need heroes to counter the villains, a Dr. Restoration who may temper the need for hasty contracts with Dr. Absolute.

I had both a medical doctor and a psychiatrist recognize CFIDS as a physiological entity separate from depression. Also, watching my family members suffer from depression, I could effectively say that CFIDS was profoundly different. I became sick with CFIDS very suddenly, with a disabling viral onset following two months of strange vertigo. Even when I tried to tell myself I was "just depressed," I knew full well that I was dealing with an entirely different and unbelievable catastrophe. To the untrained eye, CFIDS may look like a state of inflicted lethargy or dysthymia, but in reality, it feels more like an awful surreal flu that never goes away. But I did have a remarkable turning point when I found effective antidepressants to treat my own mood disorder. One day, about three weeks into my treatment protocol with the new drugs, I found myself driving along in my car, grooving to Aretha Franklin, and suddenly feeling a sense of mental well-being that I hadn't felt since childhood. Nonetheless, despite the alleviation of that familiar dark cloud, my CFIDS symptoms did not relent at all. It was just as difficult, most of the time, to walk up a flight of stairs, or lift my leaden body from the couch. Not because I didn't want to move, but because CFIDS was like being on a planet with double gravity. Still, with the medication and the help of my psychiatrist, I began to reconfigure my sense of self around this state of limbo. I stopped focusing so much on my escape, and more on the wispy and amorphous texture of the fog.

I have not had a day when I felt "normal" in several years. Sometimes I look at my old racing bike and feel indescribable longing. Sometimes the grief of my CFIDS losses is unbearable. But I am glad

I stuck around because often, truly, I am happier than I was before I got sick. My life consists of different pleasures, ones that coexist with my world of pain.

Illness has thrust me into a world of surprise. Many of the surprises are painful, such as the days I experience chest pains or unbearable chills or fevers or consuming mental confusion. But with surprise as my new dictum, I live with childlike wonder, and I relish the surprises that are good. I am not afraid of pain or grief because they weave through my days, and every day I must exhibit courage, and every day I see where my courage lives. With this, I have stopped viewing happiness and pleasure as acquisitions, but as part of my daily barometer. I lie on my back and strum chords on my new electric guitar, knowing that if I weather this illness, I will certainly have the grit and determination to be anything I want, including a stage musician. I know every lump in my pillow. I know how to cherish the good friends who *did* stick by me. I am thankful for healers who understand.

But most of all, I no longer view my life as a state of transit. I am in no hurry. I realize now that the limbo, the in-between, the transit, *is* life. Many healthy people seem to have no awareness of this. I realize that small moments of gratitude make life real. I have felt the beatific splendor of an IV drip after being wracked with chills and high fever and rushed to the emergency room. I have fumbled ecstatically into the arms of a lover just hours after finding myself in an incomprehensible, painful agony I thought would never end. I have noticed the way my dog relishes wind. A shiatsu practitioner has made my skin sink under his thumbs and called upon me to occupy every Gaza strip, every embattled zone, of my flesh. I have learned that, fundamentally, this is my body, and my life. And I will never take it for granted again, because I took so much for granted before I got sick.

This is my life. I say this mantra to myself a lot because, though many of us disbelieve it at times, we only have what we have. And what we have is a physical landscape that may be a dramatic seismic fault zone, or a place where a growing mountain is barely detectable. Either way, change is happening. And hopefully for the maligned and ignored patients with CFIDS, in a world that is just starting to have a firmer grasp on our challenges and medical needs, things can only get better.

NOTES

1. "Fibromyalgia Patient Turns to Kevorkian." *The CFIDS Chronicle,* May/June 1998, p. 12.

2. Sexton, Anne. "Wanting to Die." *The Complete Poems.* Boston: Houghton Mifflin, 1981, p. 142.

3. Schmidt, Patti. "Assisted Suicide and CFIDS: Curren Death Spurs Raging Debate." *The CFIDS Chronicle,* Fall 1996, p. 7.

4. Kenney, K. Kimberly."Doctors Share Treatment Insights: Domestic Abuse a Concern." *The CFIDS Chronicle,* November/December 1998, p. 27.

5. "CFIDS News Briefs: Patient's Suicide Linked to Kevorkian." *The CFIDS Chronicle,* Summer 1997, p. 10.

6. "AACFS Conference 1998: Psychiatric Aspects." *The CFIDS Chronicle,* January/February 1999, p. 16.

7. Berne, Katrina. "Ruling Out Depression." In *Running on Empty.* Alameda, CA: Hunter House, 1995, pp. 49-51.

8. "Dr. Gurwitt Denounces Automatic Psychiatric Referrals." *The CFIDS Chronicle,* January/February 1999, p. 24.

9. Crean, Elizabeth A. "Patients Speak Out!" *The CFIDS Chronicle,* January/February 1999, p. 26.

10. "Reduced Blood Volume Targeted." *The CFIDS Chronicle,* May/June 1998, p. 21.

Chapter 18

From Activist to "Passivist": Where Is the Mass Movement?

June Stein

"Tell me!" I demanded into the receiver, even though I already knew. I'd seen it on Channels 4 and 7; taped it off Channel 25. I played it again and again, before I got the phone call, feeling my face as I watched others' faces forced to the asphalt, as a man with a bloody gash on his forehead talked to reporters. Sitting in front of the TV, I wished I could be there in person to help wipe away the blood.

Each Thanksgiving mourners gather at Plymouth Rock. Twenty-nine years, not one Thanksgiving missed. Indians hold this National Day of Mourning because European colonists stole land and murdered millions. Because current conditions facing indigenous peoples are atrocious. Because genocide isn't easily forgotten. Speeches, marches, protest actions: one year they buried Plymouth Rock; one year some-one, who knows who, painted it blood red. In 1997, the year I tried to go but failed, the blood was real.

"The cops came at us with horses," Steve told me when he called. "They pinned us to the ground, even pepper-sprayed kids."

"You okay?" I asked. He was my only boyfriend, after all.

"Yeah. They arrested Moonanum and Mahtowin, too. Zeroed in on the leaders: twenty-five arrests—all because we had no permit to march," Steve said. "We were charged with unlawful assembly and assaulting police. Geesh. *They* beat on peaceful protesters."

I stared at the placard I'd made the night before. "Teach the Truth" it read, because I hated the good-Pilgrim-savage-Indian myth. I'd been so disappointed that morning when, weak, dizzy, I realized I was too sick to go. Yet another day chronic fatigue syndrome would win.

Others with "bigger" disabilities—folks with wheelchairs, crutches —they'd go. But I was too weak to even brush my hair. How had I made it *eight years* with this illness?

That day I had turned on the radio every hour on the hour. "Police, protesters clash in Plymouth."

Yeah? Yeah? And?

Finally that evening, after watching and taping the TV news, I got details. "It was an armed camp of cops," Steve said via phone. "Town, state, even Feds. Hundreds of 'em. . . ."

"How many of you?" I asked.

"Hundreds!"

Great. I had missed the protest of the decade.

I went to the kitchen, boiled two moldy potatoes, added powdered milk, and searched for the butter cube I'd swiped from the take-out deli the day before.

"Every inch of this land is Indian land. We don't need a permit to march on Indian land," Moonanum said on the late night news. I sat watching, eating my makeshift Thanksgiving dinner of salty mashed potatoes and frozen peas. The director of the Massachusetts ACLU said of the police's conduct: "Completely unnecessary. . . . Pretty brutal." He promised to arrange legal defense for the marchers.

Too exhausted to wash my plate, I went to bed.

My life didn't used to be like this. It used to be that I not only attended activist events, but I helped organize them. This wasn't simply because it was important and necessary work, but also because activism was in my genes. I grew up watching my parents dedicate their lives to social change. Full, intense human beings, my parents were in constant motion. They had ideas and they acted on them. They had energy and they used it. When they finally sat down, it was with others to discuss the world's injustices and to plan their next move: how to make an impact. They were idealists guided by principles lodged securely in the gut. They believed a person, once conscious of truths and injustices, would want to join the struggle. This led them to lead. They were always in front of groups of people talking, directing, teaching—initiating action. The antiwar movement, fighting racism, advocating for civil rights and gay liberation, and of course working to end women's oppression. Though in the end they focused primarily on feminism, they were initially part of all those struggles. And starting at age five I got to watch and absorb their whirlwind of activities.

Equipped with my parents' dual gifts of activist skills and a sense of empowerment, I became involved as a child and young adult in a wide variety of campaigns for social justice and social change. Perhaps it started at age ten. That was when I decided that I was not just the daughter of feminist leaders but a girl feminist in my own right. I set out to teach and lead other girls. I passed around *Ms.* magazine and *Our Bodies, Ourselves,* lectured fellow students and teachers about language (firefighters, not fire*men!*), and enrolled my best friend in fifth grade—who was being abused at home—in a self-defense course for women (at the time, this was the cutting-edge thing in the women's movement). And as I grew, my activism did too; as a young adult I founded an organization aimed at ending sexist and racist imagery in the media, led workshops on female empowerment, and organized training sessions on dismantling all *isms.* I even got a graduate degree in peace studies and climbed my way into a career—positioned with promise both for the field and myself.

Then I got sick.

I was twenty-five when I got a bad case of the flu. Six months later, I was still having difficulty getting out of bed. Soon after, I was diagnosed with CFIDS. That was when I discovered the truth about my activism. All my life I had been holding on to the erroneous belief—a belief held by every cell in my body—that my self-worth was tied to making a difference in the world. I felt that I must always be actively working to right wrongs or I was not doing enough, as though *I* was not enough. I suppose at first glance, to a healthy, able-bodied person, this mind-set might not seem like such a bad thing. But after experiencing a chronic illness that kept me nearly bedridden and disabled for years, and watching my self-esteem plummet at the same rate as my activist abilities, I now know that having one's self-worth so intricately tied to being an active force for change is not good.

Even after nine years with this illness, I continue to grieve over my inability to get out and try to change the world for the better. And when I can, I still do dedicate my time and energy to social causes, including CFIDS activism. But this is minimal. Less than minimal. Practically nothing. It seems that every time I try to initiate a real project or activity, more than just writing a letter of complaint to the National Institutes of Health, I am cut down by brain fog, weak limbs, and an inability to push past an unrelenting exhaustion that feels not unlike an elephant sitting on my poor crushed body.

In this state of constant illness, the former activist in me, the woman usually so prone to organizing and seeking positive change, wants to ask: is this exhaustion, body pain, and fog what has kept all of us PWCs (People with CFIDS) from forming an aggressive nation-wide CFIDS movement—or is there something more?

Certainly there are dedicated individuals and even organizations that have fought the good fight for CFIDS patients for the past decade and a half. They have been on the forefront of the battle to get our illness recognized as legitimate, to get doctors and researchers to focus on both a cause and cure, and to get the government to take our needs seriously. And these advocates and activists deserve our deeply felt thanks and appreciation.

But really, besides these few individuals and organizations, where has the *mass* movement been? About 800,000 people in this country alone have CFIDS. With those kinds of numbers, why haven't we—why haven't I—taken to the streets? Or at the very least, why haven't we flooded our federal representatives' offices with weekly letters and visits demanding both recognition and research money? Even the sickest of us could write weekly letters. Likely 50 percent of us could make the trip to our local representative's office to meet with a legislative aide. And certainly more of us could get to the annual May 12 Washington, DC, National Lobbying Day than have made it in previous years. At the very least, once, just once, why haven't a few of us stood outside the Centers for Disease Control with placards that say, "Where'd our money go?" (Author's note: this is making reference to a top CDC official's [William Reeves] 1997 whistle-blowing acknowledgment that millions of congressionally allocated dollars, originally dedicated to CFIDS, were illegally misspent, thereby never making it to CFIDS-related research. Reeves also said his superiors lied about this misspending to Congress.) And everyone has heard the joke about holding a "sleep-in" on the steps of the U.S. Capitol. In our pajamas. The idea might give us all a good chuckle, but it would likely get great media coverage, thus making it a viable tactic.

So, what is it that keeps us, including me, from organizing more aggressively? Why haven't we been able to form, like the community of people with HIV, an ACT UP-type of organization, the organization that wisely made such an in-your-face stink that AIDS was finally, belatedly, put on the U.S. government and media's radar screen?

In answering these questions I can only speak for myself. First, I don't want to underestimate the degree to which I am physically disabled and how that prevents my activism. From what I can tell, from the moment I got this illness I was as sick as some of the individuals I have heard about who were suffering from the mid-to-late stages of AIDS. I was close to bedridden for years. Taking a shower was too taxing. Brushing my teeth, too exhausting. If I was able to take a miniwalk one day, or get my butt to the doctor's office, I paid for it for the next three. Getting to a single protest planning meeting would have been impossible. If I could change from my nighttime PJ's to daytime sweats, I considered the day a success. I had gone from activist to "passivist" because I was too sick to ACT UP.

And there is another angle to this AIDS-versus-CFIDS degree of disability. It used to be, in ACT UP's heyday, that getting HIV was a death sentence. Getting CFIDS was (is) not. I can only assume that knowing someone who might die energizes and activates that person and his or her family. For me, getting CFIDS, the flight was not to the streets but rather to retreat. Actually, I had no choice. Suddenly my body was doing strange things, like finding it hard to walk, or even stand up. Suddenly I couldn't trust my mind to think of the right words, or find the proper left turn that would lead to my house, even though I had taken the same route home a thousand times before. Everything in my world was turned upside down. I was scared. Besides, suddenly I found that my former joy in life—interacting with people—became too exhausting, even by phone. My first priority became energy conservation.

Part of my flight, my withdrawing from the world, was due to my second priority: research—finding something that would get me out of the new horror I faced. I used what scraps of energy I could conjure up to find treatments, doctors, a mattress I could tolerate, a shampoo that wouldn't make my now chemically sensitive self pass out from its smelly perfume. Needing to retreat from big things was understandable; but even little things became too much. Listening to the radio, reading the newspaper: the stimulation was overwhelming. In isolation and seclusion, with no stimuli—this became the only way I could live.

And far from an HIV/AIDS death sentence (as it used to be, still is for some, but thankfully no longer is the norm, if only in wealthy Western countries), everyone in my family assumed I'd be better in a few months' time. I did, too. We all thought I just had to wait it out. And though sometimes I felt like I was going to die, and sometimes it got so bad I even *wished* I would die, I wasn't going to. No, I just had to live under house arrest—chained to the bed, detained, literally incarcerated by an inexplicable bodily collapse. One year passed. Then two. It was years into the illness before I understood that I *could* have this for a long time, perhaps my whole life. And it was years after that realization when I finally came out of denial and saw that unless there was some medical breakthrough I *would* have this for life. (And like a delayed reaction, my family is still having trouble coming out of their denial. They still can't believe I will be sick for the rest of my life.) In short, I moved from assuming I certainly *would* get better and get my life back at some point in time, to assuming I would *not* get better, and that I'd better start building a new life, as a disabled person. I applied for Social Security Disability and cried for two weeks straight.

However, things changed. As the years went by I got more energy. I can now, irregularly, and only on unpredictable days, sit and write at my computer like a "normal" person for a few hours at a time. Now I can do my own food shopping. Now I can talk on the phone without getting exhausted. Now I can definitively say that I am only bedridden 25 percent of the time—with occasional, unpredictable bouts, which last indefinitely (months, even), of being bedridden 100 percent of the time. In other words, it is still hell. For example, last year I made it to a one-week writers' workshop. But then I got a bad relapse and spent the next six months in bed, watching every *Simpsons* show in syndication.

In my current state, it is this very unpredictability that has kept me from activism. The few times I did try to either initiate an activist event, or simply partake in one, I would work for a few days on a project and then get "hit." I'd crawl back to bed for weeks, months—cursing myself for ever having been optimistic, for dashing my and other people's hopes of pulling off the planned fundraiser/educational initiative/organizing endeavor. A strong aversion to even *trying* to get active in CFIDS activism set in.

Clearly, my physical state is still keeping me from hitting the streets with protesting placards. But is there more, besides a physical disability that keeps me—us—from forming a more aggressive CFIDS movement? Sure is. You need economic resources to mount a serious campaign. Living on a Social Security Disability check gives me $475 per month. After food, rent—there's not a whole heck of a lot there to work with.

Okay, but what about simply organizing a massive letter-writing campaign? Each year on May 12 we try, and succeed, in getting some attention. But what about even *more* letters? What about *every* 12th of *each* month? I mean, there are 800,000 of us. Is there some reason we haven't done even this? Some reason *I* haven't?

Yes—only the answer is a lot less tangible than lack of money. It is an emotional state that has blocked me (us?)—and it can be summed up in three quick words: abandonment, disappointment, despair. But it took me a while to settle into those three words, and in that interim I first had to accumulate a whole lot of emotional burnout.

And from where does this burnout arise, you might ask?

Try years of explaining my invisible symptoms to a society that just didn't buy it. Basically, every day I had to defend my credibility. The lack of legitimacy surrounding CFIDS came from a media who deemed my hellish reality a mere "yuppie flu" and a government who flat-out denied its existence. This took a toll. I began the arduous task of proving myself. Over and over again, for nine years, I have been trying to convince others that though my cheeks are pink and rosy, though my body still has all its limbs, I am horribly sick and in fact quite disabled. I have given the *I know I look fine but really I am very, very, sick and spend half my existence bedridden* speech literally thousands of times. Each time I hope I get the understanding nod, not the dreaded squinting of disbelieving eyes. Each eye squint cuts away at my self-esteem. Cuts away at my ability to trust myself. *Maybe I am not really sick. I mean, yesterday I* was *able to go food shopping and still cook dinner after that.*

Forget the fact that I had spent the two months prior unable to have friends visit for even an hour because it was too exhausting.

But I can't help questioning my own illness when everyone around me does, too. And the fact is that there is no known cause and no known "marker" to definitively identify which of us has the illness. Thrown into this suspicion-creating cauldron is the confusing reality that some of us, like me, have "good" days—times when I am able to be up and about. Those days are great because I can make it to the post office and get my car oil changed, but they are also tainted by a nagging inner doubt. Those are the days I am more likely to buy into the skepticism I feel around me, more likely to think, *Maybe I'm not really. . . .*

A suspicious public, continually trying to prove myself, and inner battles with self-doubt: an exhausting mix, even for a healthy body! But this is not all that has brought on the emotional burnout I feel. Add the fact that the government—our government, the one we pay taxes to, the one that is to serve and protect us—is at *best* guilty of negligence and at *worst* guilty of purposeful betrayal. They denied my illness existed for years and then, with chilling premeditation, illegally misspent funds for medical research that could have helped to give me back my life—years ago. Years ago!

The government is not the only one who has no interest in me and feels no sense of responsibility. The media, too. For years it has ignored published, peer-reviewed medical research on my illness. It ignored a 1996 public letter from Assistant Secretary of Health and Human Services Philip Lee about the seriousness of CFIDS. Lee sent his letter to all the national newspapers. Not one published nor covered it in an article. Similarly, in 1998, when William Reeves, the CDC official in charge of CFIDS, came forward under the government's whistle-blower act and asserted that millions of dollars of CFIDS funds were misspent, and when it became clear that CDC officials might have lied to Congress about it, no major media outlets wanted to run a story on it. My friends and I called/faxed/e-mailed numerous news outlets. Nothing. It was like I didn't exist. Like the major struggle of my life was a nonissue. And even when the U.S. Inspector General's report came out, confirming the allegations of misspent monies, the media barely yawned. Yes, there were a few articles in a few national publications, but was the response proportionate to the outrageous act—the alleged illegal act? Was there any media call for heads to roll? No.

Sometimes it feels like even those rare few who *are* trying to help PWCs—like the CFIDS medical researchers —have also abandoned me. Medical researchers, by definition, have something the government and media would respect: knowledge and credibility. And what do they do with it? *Research*, of all things. I have often wondered, watching the same *Simpsons* rerun for the tenth time, too beat to do anything else—*Wouldn't their time be better spent taking a stand as vocal advocates for PWCs?* Instead, researchers work to keep a steady flow of money coming, to keep their research projects going. Yes, yes, I appreciate it, but if not from them, where will our spokespersons, our voice of credibility, come from?

Certainly not the CFIDS community. We are too busy infighting. Hillary Johnson's excellent book, *Osler's Web,* magnified the splinters that already existed in the CFIDS community. There are two camps: those who want to work with the government and those who perceive the government as the enemy. There is a lack of consensus, bickering, name-calling. When we are so busy fighting among ourselves, who on the outside will bother to listen to us or perceive us as having any legitimacy?

Coupled with my sense of abandonment is that truly delightful feeling of *disappointment.* Having CFIDS is a study in disappointment. Besides being majorly disappointed that I don't get to have my life, as I had expected I would (as everyone expects they will), I am also challenged by daily mini-disappointments. Oh, guess I won't be going to my best friend's wedding. Can't drive. Oh, guess I won't be going to that play I already bought tickets for. Can't sit up for two hours. Oh, guess I won't make it to the library today. The lights, the mold, the people. Hi-ho, hi-ho, it's off to bed I go. They should call it chronic disappointment syndrome.

Disappointment also comes from experiencing perpetually built up and then dashed hopes. Every few months I hear of a supposed breakthrough: new reports (that most in the medical community seem to ignore) on causes, treatments, diagnostic markers, cures. Neurally mediated hypotension, Florinef, low blood volume, mycoplasma, intensive antibiotic therapy, mitochondrial dysfunction, Neurontin. Standing chest-deep in a cool pool? Magnetic mattresses? Desperate people do desperate things. I've tried them all. Rarely do I find anything that works. In fact, most new treatments make me worse. How long can I ride this roller coaster of high hopes followed by deep disappointments? Neither, though, can I avoid it. Because without a sense of hope . . . well, let's just say that those without hope don't make it to the next day of *Simpsons* reruns. It is a tightrope balancing act, a fine line: holding onto the hope of finding something that will help, and yet still accepting my disabled reality—and moving on with my new, albeit hard to accept, life. I succeed in this balancing act; I am there each day at 6:00 p.m. to watch Bart and Lisa Simpson. But I also can't help falling, regularly, into the net of despair positioned under my tightrope.

The year after I missed the 1997 National Day of Mourning at Plymouth Rock, about a month before Thanksgiving 1998, Steve called. He was no longer my boyfriend, but still able to make me smile: "Sometimes disaster turns to victory," he said. "The town settled!"

The Indian-led boycott, letter-writing campaign (which included four letters from me), and the defendants' suit against police for excessive force worked. The Town of Plymouth, Massachusetts, dropped all charges against the protesters.

Even better, Steve said, now and forever on the Day of Mourning Indians can march without a permit. And they'll march by two new monuments erected by the town; one of King Philip, a Wampanoag leader who battled English settlers stealing Indian land, and one commemorating the Day of Mourning itself. My favorite part of the settlement was that Plymouth will also give money to "Teach the Truth" to school kids, about our country's history of genocide and the historic blood on Plymouth Rock.

All this meant that 1998's Day of Mourning was also going to be, in some sense, a victory party. And I wanted to be there. So in 1998, though now wondering how I had survived *nine years* of illness, though still too disabled to do the hour drive by myself, though still too weak to properly have my hair brushed, I made it. And even if I hadn't, I would still have felt good in knowing that my letters had, in some small way, helped to tip the scales. When you have CFIDS you not only learn to accept the daily mini-disappointments, but you also learn to celebrate the mini-contributions that lead to mini, and major, victories.

Chapter 19

The Gulf War's Troubling Legacy

Gary Null

With only 148 Americans officially killed in action and only 467 wounded, ours seemed to be a shining victory in the Gulf. But this victory has lost its glow somewhat, now that we know that tens of thousands of our Gulf service people have become sick from a debilitating and sometimes deadly syndrome. According to H. Lindsey Arison III, aide to the undersecretary of the U.S. Air Force, there are now 50,000 veterans suffering from Gulf War syndrome, including about 11,000 on active duty.[1]

Arison outlines the causes of Gulf vets' health problems. First, they were exposed to nonlethal levels of chemical and biological agents released primarily by direct Iraqi attack via missiles, rockets, artillery, or aircraft munitions and by fallout from allied bombings of Iraqi chemical warfare munitions facilities during the thirty-eight-day 1991 war.

Exposure to chemical and biological agents alone is one thing. But the effects of these were exacerbated by a whole gamut of other factors to which vets were exposed. Arison enumerates them: nerve agent pretreatment pills that our service people were ordered to take; investigational botulinum toxoid vaccines; anthrax vaccines; and depleted uranium, used in armor-piercing munitions. Other factors enter into the synergistic mix including oil fire contamination and pesticides, and some people believe that an artificially engineered bacterium/virus cross called a mycoplasma, and, separately, that a vaccine ingredient, the adjuvant squalene, were significant factors, too.

"The Gulf War's Troubling Legacy" originally appeared, in a much longer form, in *The Townsend Letter,* August/September 1998, and October 1998. Excerpted with permission.

Arison emphasizes the point that since different people were exposed to different hazards at different levels, a whole variety of symptomatologies have arisen in Gulf War vets. This variability of symptoms is sometimes taken to mean that Gulf War syndrome is a "mystery illness" or that people are imagining things, when in fact it just shows that the syndrome is a multifactorial problem.

SYMPTOMS

Gulf War syndrome (GWS) is manifested in many ways. Chronic fatigue immune dysfunction syndrome (CFIDS) affects over half of the victims, according to Dr. Garth Nicolson, who, with his wife, molecular biophysicist and University of Texas professor Dr. Nancy Nicolson, has examined and evaluated many syndrome patients.[2] Public health expert Dr. Leonard Horwitz estimates that 80 to 90 percent of syndrome patients are plagued with severe aches and pains in their joints.[3] Others commonly experience dizziness, nausea, stomach pains, light sensitivity, intense anxiety, breathing difficulty, muscle spasms, diarrhea, blurred vision, inexplicable skin rashes, bleeding gums, eye redness, night sweats, and acute migraine-like headaches. Sexual and urination disorders plague numerous victims, and 25 percent have acquired multiple chemical sensitivities, which means they have become allergic to a wide variety of chemical substances and can consequently have severe reactions to even the most common household items.

According to Drs. Garth and Nancy Nicolson, the CFIDS characteristic of sick Gulf vets is induced by an unusual microorganism that seems to be the product of weaponization, that is, human manipulation of germs for the purposes of warfare.[4] The Nicolsons report that the organism present in each of the CFIDS patients is an odd variant of a typical mycoplasma. Ordinarily, a mycoplasma is a cross between a bacterium and a virus, and can be effectively combated with antibiotics. But in this case, the organism contains human immunodeficiency virus (HIV-1) and anthrax genes. Since it is not possible for the typical mycoplasma to naturally mutate into a modified form of anthrax and the alleged AIDS virus, this seems to be an engineered organism. The Nicolsons contend that the U.S. military created this mycoplasma and sold it to Iraq, which subsequently used it against U.S. troops.

UNPROVEN VACCINES, UNMONITORED MEDICINE

The widespread use of experimental vaccines during Desert Storm has often been cited as a possible cause of Gulf War syndrome. Dr. Garth Nicolson elaborates: "I'm not a big fan of experimental vaccines. There have been too many mistakes."[5] He explains that during the Gulf War, the established procedures of vaccination were ignored. Normally, only one inoculation should be given at a time, but the military insisted on giving multiple shots at once, which, according to Nicolson, is the worst thing you can do because it suppresses the immune system.

The troops immunized for the Gulf have been called guinea pigs, and for good reason. They received experimental vaccines, e.g., those for anthrax and botulinum that were not approved for use by the FDA and have since proven to cause potentially dangerous side effects. Because of these vaccines' experimental nature, many questions have arisen as to why our government dispensed them. Not the least of these questions is, what about the Nuremberg Code? Developed by the Allies after World War II in response to inhumane Nazi experimentation, the Nuremberg Code says that *voluntary and informed consent is absolutely essential from all human subjects who participate in research, whether during peace or war.*

Nerve-gas-countering pills were a big problem for many Desert Storm participants. Documents released by the Pentagon in 1995 revealed that high-ranking military officials had pressured the Food and Drug Administration into authorizing experimentation with pyridostigmine bromide (PB) tablets for protection against Iraqi chemical or biological attacks. PB tablets are usually only used for the treatment of the chronic muscle weakness disorder called myasthenia gravis, but the military and the FDA waived the traditional informed consent procedures during the early stages of the conflict. Many soldiers did inquire about the classified nature of the pills, but, nevertheless, they were forced to consume them in excessive quantities by their commanding officers. Others, fearing for their safety, ignored the orders of their superiors after witnessing the pills' highly unpleasant gastric effects upon their fellow service members.

WHERE WAS THE FDA?

Isn't the FDA responsible for making sure that Americans aren't given unsafe drugs? Shouldn't they at least warn people of possible dangers? They claim they tried. They blame the Pentagon for PB. In May 1997, it was reported that a top FDA official told Congress the Pentagon did not keep a promise to fully inform soldiers before giving them the experimental nerve gas antidotes during the war.[6] The promise to warn soldiers about the drugs had been a condition of the FDA's agreeing, in 1991, to waive standard consent requirements. A Pentagon spokesperson said that information sheets had been sent to the Gulf, but sent late. Some members of Congress were outraged upon hearing this. For instance, Christopher Shays (R.–Connecticut), chairman of the congressional investigating committee, said that the FDA's failure to compel the military to keep its word "blows my mind."

Evidence has indicated that the procedure for administering the pills placed the recipients at risk. Records of who received the pills were not kept, and a standard dosage was distributed, regardless of sex, age, weight, or medical history. What's more, the toxicity of this experimental drug was actually heightened by issuing it along with common household insecticides, a potentially lethal combination.

IRAQ'S DEADLY ARSENAL

Another possible cause of Gulf War syndrome was the presence of biological and chemical additives present in the Scud B and Frog missiles. On May 1, 1996, senior physician at Walter Reed Army Hospital Major General Ronald Blanck admitted to the President's Panel on Gulf War Illnesses that chemical and biological weapons had been used during Operation Desert Storm, and that low-level exposures to these agents probably occurred. Studies have confirmed that hundreds of Iraqi missiles had been loaded with biological warfare agents, but until Major General Blanck's report—five years after the war—the evidence had been completely disavowed by official sources.

Disclosures by high-ranking Iraqi officials have in fact confirmed that Iraq possessed an extensive chemical and biological arsenal during the Gulf War. After the August 1995 defection of Lieutenant General

Hussein Kamel Majid, Saddam Hussein's top biological weapons adviser, the Iraqi government, in an attempt to lessen the impact of Majid's revelations, unveiled an abundance of classified information to United Nations investigators documenting the development of biological and chemical warfare arsenals.[7]

The Iraqis revealed that prior to the Gulf War their nation engaged in a top secret program to develop biological, chemical, and nuclear weapons that could be used against any of their foes, including the United States, Israel, and Saudi Arabia. Prior to the disclosures, Iraq had claimed that it had only ten people employed at its biological programs, but it has since admitted that 150 scientists and an extensive support staff were involved in the mass development of biological warfare agents in the 1980s. According to the UN officials, Iraq possessed at least fifty bombs loaded with anthrax, one hundred bombs containing botulinum, and twenty-five missile warheads carrying other germ agents.[8]

THE UNITED STATES AS SUPPLIER
OF CHEMICAL WEAPONS

A sad irony of the Gulf War involves the origin of Iraq's biological and chemical weapons. At least some of them came from the United States. By sharing weapons and intelligence throughout Iraq's long war with Iran in the 1980s, the United States helped create the largest stockpile of chemical weapons in history. That these were later used to our detriment is an example of the phenomenon known as "blowback," i.e., what happens when we don't look at the long-term consequences of our foreign policy actions.

According to the Riegle Report, during the 1980s the U.S. government supplied the Iraqi Atomic Energy Commission with at least twenty-eight biological weapons to use in its bitter war with neighboring Iran.[9] In 1987, then Vice President Bush met with Iraqi officials to ensure that technological equipment used to produce chemical and biological warfare agents would continue to be exported to the Iraqis. When he assumed the presidency, Bush maintained this policy, despite congressional dissension. Corporations involved in transactions with the Iraqi government, including Hewlett-Packard, Honeywell, Rockwell, and Tektronix, were licensed to export more than $1.5 million of highly sophisticated equipment in the five years preceding the Gulf War, and these companies frequently delivered their products directly to Iraqi chemical and nuclear plants.

In his report to Congress, Senator Riegle was quite explicit, being able to name the biologicals involved, the batch numbers sent to Iraq, and their dates. For instance, among the agents delivered to various agencies of the Iraqi government were *Clostridium perfringens,* a gaseous gangrene-causing agent, *Brucella melitensis, Clostridium botulinum, Salmonella, Klebsiella pneumoniae, Escherichia coli, Bacillus subtilis,* and *Staphylococcus epidermidis.*[10]

The United States was a participant in the Geneva Biological Weapons Convention of 1972, and we (as well as Iraq!) signed the resultant agreement that prohibited both experimentation with and the sale of biologicals or weapons of mass destruction. Now, obviously, our government has a considerable interest in keeping the U.S. breach of this agreement covered up. Plus, there's the inconvenient fact of our history of cooperation with Saddam Hussein, a tyrant who was denounced by the global community and likened to Adolf Hitler. Embarrassment about revealing our past dealings with our current enemy has hampered our government's readiness to deal fairly with veterans.

UNHEEDED ALARMS

Many Gulf War veterans have testified that chemical warfare detector alarms at bases across the region were frequently triggered, yet troops were ordered to ignore the alarms. According to General Colin Powell, who had been chairman of the Joint Chiefs of Staff during the war, American commanders had believed the frequent alarms to be false, because nobody seemed to be getting sick immediately.[11] It was believed by those involved that one had to become obviously ill at the time of exposure to chemical or biological agents for exposure to mean anything.

A HALF-DECADE OF COVER-UP

From 1991 to 1996, the Pentagon basically took a see-no-evil approach regarding the causes of Gulf War syndrome. In a document titled "Memorandum for Persian Gulf Veterans," released on May 25, 1994, Defense Secretary William Perry and Joint Chiefs of Staff chairman General John Shalikashvili assured veterans that there was no evidence, classified or unclassified, suggesting that chemical or biological weapons were used in the Gulf,[12] while a June 23, 1994, report by the Pentagon's science board attempted to reinforce that argument, asserting that service members were not exposed to chemical or biological elements at any level.[13]

THE PENTAGON BEGINS TO COME CLEAN

It was at a Washington press conference on June 21, 1996, that the Pentagon finally began to drop its know-nothing stance. They admitted that the demolition of an Iraqi ammunition depot, just after the war's end, may have released chemical agents, including mustard gas and sarin. According to Defense Department officials, United Nations inspectors who had visited the site at the Kamisiyah ammunition depot in southern Iraq in May 1996 had verified traces of these deadly gases at the ruins of a bunker destroyed in March 1991. At the press conference, Pentagon spokesperson Kenneth Bacon also admitted that documentation of this incident had existed as early as 1991, but that it had been temporarily misplaced in the abundance of Pentagon paperwork. The lost-paperwork excuse, though, was all too familiar.

ARE GULF VETS REALLY SICKER?

For years now, there has been the idea that while Gulf War syndrome illnesses may exist, they're really an old problem—a response to stress—with a new name, and that Gulf veterans are in reality no sicker than other vets. But in November 1996, the chairwoman of a federal panel investigating the issue contended that Gulf conflict participants are in fact sicker than other soldiers. Prominent toxicologist Eula Bingham concluded that, clearly, Gulf vets were suffering from a disproportionate level of ailments.[14] One of the reasons this had been unclear probably had to do with what investigators were looking at. While government reports had shown that our Gulf troops were not dying or falling seriously ill at disproportionate rates, many of the vets' ailments—such as gastrointestinal symptoms, chronic fatigue, and aching joints—do not usually result in what researchers had been looking for—hospitalization or early death. Thus, the vets' symptoms were not taken into proper account.

THE POWER OF SYNERGY

More and more truths are being acknowledged about the Gulf War syndrome picture, and one of the most important is that our troops were exposed not just to a single toxin, but to a whole variety. So we can't lose sight of the power of synergy. That is, when two or more relatively weak illness-causing factors are combined, they can be quite harmful. This was underscored by a January 1997 paper by researchers who had studied both experimental animals and Gulf War vets at the University of Texas Southwestern Medical Center in Dallas. Their findings: Harmless levels of two or more chemicals can combine to cause precisely the symptoms reported by Gulf War syndrome sufferers. These symptoms appear to be a type of organophosphate poisoning, report the researchers. What's more, they note that the subtle nerve damage caused by organophosphate poisoning can be missed by physicians unfamiliar with the phenomenon.[15]

Additional work done at the Southwestern Medical Center shows stronger evidence that chemical synergy—not stress—is what's making vets sick. Professor of clinical neurology Jim Hom was a principal investigator on this study. He explained that the researchers compared a broad range of brain-related psychological functions of ill and well veterans from the Twenty-Fourth Naval Mobile Construction Battalion. The scientists were blinded as to which group was which until the end of the work.[16]

"The ill veterans performed worse on 59 of the 71 brain-related measures," Hom reported, adding that the affected vets' psychological profile was similar to that of individuals with general medical problems and did not include psychopathology. "Clearly, the ill veterans demonstrated a neuropsychological pattern of impairment that is indicative of generalized brain damage, not psychological reactions."[17]

What was particularly noteworthy about Hom's study was that it refuted the results of an earlier study done at the Birmingham VA

Medical Center by researchers who used many, but not all, of the same neuropsychological tests. In that study, fifty-five Gulf vets with cognitive difficulties were tested, and the VA researchers concluded that exposure to neurotoxins did not come into play, attributing the vets' symptoms to "intentional exaggeration of problems" or "emotional distress," and going as far as to say that some of the vets were faking.

But there was a problem with the Birmingham study, Hom explained: It had no control group. The Dallas study, by contrast, had a control group of veterans from the same unit who were not reporting any problems. "When you stack all the results of our tests together it is clear that something is wrong. The brain is an organ that integrates all types of functions. You can't isolate and test just one thing. The tests have to be complementary. Our tests were designed to be a package—they complemented each other. This is what makes our study different from others."

Commented Hom's co-researcher Dr. Robert Haley, "This study supports our overall theory that the syndrome we identified represents neurological damage from combinations of chemicals."

And Hom said, when asked about the psychological aspects of Gulf War syndrome, "Psychological issues are important—but they don't cause brain damage."

STRONG INSECTICIDES USED

Hom and Haley's studies, as well as others done recently with Duke University scientists, are finally demonstrating that chemical synergy, rather than combat stress, is the underlying factor in Gulf War syndrome. Because of all the toxins to which troops were exposed—including pesticides; insect repellent, sometimes used in the form of flea collars worn by soldiers, and including DEET; nerve gas; anti-nerve gas medication; experimental vaccines; burning oil-well fumes; and depleted uranium—the potential for synergistic damage is extensive, and hard to fully comprehend.

Use of insect repellent is a mundane factor that nevertheless ought not to be overlooked when considering synergistic damage. *Stars and Stripes* reports that while the insecticide DEET was deemed safe in concentrations of less than 31 percent, Desert Storm participants received DEET in strengths between 33 and 75 percent.[18] The combination of DEET and PB—those pyridostigmine bromide anti-nerve gas pills that servicemen and women were ordered to take—is being studied at the University of Florida at Gainesville for their combined effects. Also, the insecticide permethrin, sprayed on soldiers' uniforms, was used in strengths exceeding safe levels, and may have exacerbated the effects of other substances.

WHY WE NEED TO LEARN MORE

There is still a lot to understand about our Gulf experience and its aftermath. One field of inquiry involves Garth Nicolson's contention that a genetically altered mycoplasma is responsible for some Gulf War illness. Another centers on the role of depleted uranium. And an emerging question involves the Kamisiyah arms depot demolition.

One of the most important questions that will be researched is the extent to which low-level chemical exposure affects people over the long term. That there is an effect was in fact documented years ago, i.e., in a 1974 study titled "Delayed Toxic Effects of Chemical Warfare Agents."[19] This study, conducted by the director of the Institute of Chemical Toxicology of the East German Academy of Sciences, Dr. Karlbeinz Lohs, describes how workers at chemical weapons plants were diagnosed with chronic disorders that were the same as symptoms currently being exhibited by Gulf War veterans. The whole gamut of problems is the same. And further research has shown that exposure to organophosphate insecticides, which in essence are diluted forms of chemical warfare agents, can promote the onset of chronic health disorders.

In short, the evidence is there. Gulf veterans are suffering from more than stress. And as the body of current research expands upon that of the past, no one will be able to deny that truth.

NOTES

1. Arison, H. Lindsey III; personal communication, July 14, 1995.
2. Gary Null interview with Drs. Garth and Nancy Nicolson, May 7, 1996.
3. Gary Null interview with Dr. Leonard Horowitz.
4. Gary Null interview with Drs. Garth and Nancy Nicolson, May 7, 1996.

5. Ibid.

6. *Cleveland Plain Dealer,* May 9, 1997.

7. Tracy, Mary Frances, "Iraq Discloses Biological Weapons Capabilities." Posted at <http://sun00781.dn.net/news/iraq/1995/cbiacoct95.htm>.

8. Ibid.

9. Riegle, Donald W., Jr. and Alfonse M. D'Amato, "The Riegle Report: U.S. Chemical and Biological Warfare-Related Dual Use Exports to Iraq and Their Possible Impact on Health Consequences of the Gulf War." A report to the United States Senate, 103rd Congress, 2nd Session, May 25, 1994. Posted at <http://www.gulfweb.org/bigdoc/report/riegle1.html>.

10. Ibid.

11. Shenon, Philip, "Powell Says He Had No Evidence of Toxic Chemicals in Gulf War," *The New York Times,* December 3, 1996, pp. 1, 16.

12. U.S. Department of Defense, Assistant Secretary of Defense (Public Affairs), News Release No. 323-94, Department of Defense Letter of Gulf War Veterans, May 26, 1997.

13. Statement made by John Deutch, Deputy Secretary of the Department of Defense, to CBS News, *60 Minutes,* March 12, 1995.

14. Shenon, Philip, "Panel Disputes Studies on Gulf War Illness," *The New York Times,* November 21, 1996.

15. Leary, Warren E., "Gulf Illness May Reflect Multiple Exposures, Report Says," *The New York Times,* January 9, 1997, p. 18.

16. Fillmore, Randolph, "Gulf Brain Damage Report Conflicts with Earlier 'Faking' Conclusion," *Stars and Stripes,* August 25, 1997.

17. Reuters News Service, Dallas, August 1, 1997.

18. Fillmore, Randolph, "Gulf Brain Damage Report Conflicts with Earlier 'Faking' Conclusion," *Stars and Stripes,* August 25, 1997.

19. Cary, Peter and Mike Tharp, "The Gulf War's Grave Aura," *U.S. News and World Report,* July 8, 1996, pp. 33-34.

Chapter 20

The Amazing Illness
That Doesn't Exist

Chris Szabo

Not so long ago, at the time of this writing, the respected *Wall Street Journal* alleged in a prominent editorial that there was no such thing as chronic fatigue syndrome, and that CFIDS sufferers were in fact only trying to "make it much easier for people claiming to suffer from chronic fatigue [syndrome] to qualify for disability benefits."[1] Well, that most certainly couldn't have referred to me. Living in South Africa, I can safely say that, effectively, there are no Social Security benefits. And I should know.

To go back to 1993, I used up my private medical aid (which is a form of self-funded medical insurance) long before the year was over. Then came 1994. I was retrenched, with a rather small "Retrenchment Package" and was in fact very lucky to have gotten anything at all. After that, I was on my wife's medical aid. My key problem was the effective collapse of my immune system. I had been a strong, rather robust person, and could hold my own with the best of the hard-working journalists on various shifts, long hours, and extreme but invigorating work pressure. During this time, however, my company ignored doctors' letters to remove me from shifts and increased my weekly hours from 45 to 60, despite my attempts to seek help from trade unions and lawyers. After what we termed my "burnout," which also involved a long and acrimonious fight with my department head and corporation, I got sick for no reason at all. If there were a virus anywhere in Africa, it seemed, it would somehow find me. The immune antibodies IgA and IgM in my system crashed to dangerously low levels, and I got sick especially with upper respiratory tract illnesses, all of which were "opportunistic infections." I must say, I gave them plenty of "opportunity," because hardly had I finished a stomach bug, when I would get a cold, which would go to bronchitis, which would immediately go to pneumonia.

If I remember correctly, there were years when I had pneumonia four times in a row. I was given injections of Beriglobin, which replaced the missing antibodies, or immune proteins, but these were terribly expensive. Looking back, there can be no doubt that the acrimony and even brutal treatment I received at work contributed to the condition and to real stress, which led to serious problems all around. The seriousness of the issue is such that I may not name the company because, if I do, I will get slapped with a huge lawsuit aimed at totally destroying everything my wife and I have left, and would even include my father. So much for freedom of speech in the new South Africa! After a Supreme Court interdict, I found I was becoming very seriously depressed. I felt that all I understood to be true was false; that right was wrong, that a company could destroy the health of an employee and just get away with it, and that employees had no recourse to do anything at all. This shattered my faith in humanity, in God, in all my beliefs. I was diagnosed as depressed in 1995, and the psychiatrist in question said either I go on a holiday, or she would have to book me into a psychiatric hospital, and she couldn't promise when I might be able to leave, if ever.

As you can imagine, I was quite shaken by this, so I took part of the package and some savings (in those days we still had savings) and took my wife on a trip to Europe. We visited my other home, Hungary, and then Britain, where I was born and my wife's family came from. Western Europe, even Hungary, was a shock. We only realized then how far back South Africa had slipped in things like city management, road and rail transport, currency devaluation, and of course crime. In Europe (where I was born) we felt like country bumpkins. The locals would wait patiently for the lights to change; we would dash across between trucks and cars. They would expect the telephones to work, people to phone back when promised, airplanes to arrive and leave on time. When we got back, we realized that we wanted to live with the mentality in which we were brought up, with the idea that hard work is rewarded and laziness is not; and that one's qualifications matter, rather than which political party one belongs to or the color of one's skin, which we found to be too pale for the new elites.

Most people are unaware that the old, apartheid South Africa didn't only discriminate against black, brown, or yellow people. There was also "separateness" (apartheid) among whites. The top echelon were the Afrikaners; they became managers and ministers of state, regardless of ability. The next layer were the English-speaking South Africans, notably in the realm of banking and business. Next came the lowest of the white forms of life—myself—the immigrant (I came here at the age of seven).

In the new South Africa, the top echelon changed. However, tragically, the middle and bottom parts of society appeared largely unaffected, and the "heroes of the people" appeared uninterested in the poor and the needy. As for our chances in the Brave New World, they appeared unchanged, or even made worse. This had a powerful effect on our lives. Affirmative action was introduced, and soon my wife, our only support, was doing the work of an editor, but being paid the salary of a journalist. She was never told to her face to forget promotion, but it soon became clear that she could.

What has all this to do with chronic fatigue syndrome? I think a great deal. It took away much of my motivation, and I am sure that psychological stress must affect the physical, purely somatic aspects of our health. Also, we had our savings and my wife's salary to hang on to, but with my treatment paid for exclusively by us, we were looking at a bleak future indeed. As a result of both the ongoing infections and all these psychologically negative experiences, I was very ill for most of 1996. All I really did that year was write letters to people in more fortunate climes, but it kept my attention from wandering and my depression from deepening. I was put on antidepressants, but then, once we had that controlled, the ugly CFIDS showed itself clearly. My immune system began to act better, and an expert professor at the former Hillbrow Hospital in Johannesburg took me off the injections. Still, I was constantly getting flu, colds, stomach problems, and bronchopneumonias, or just bronchitis.

I can tell you, I became acquainted with the word *pain* in these years. The pain of the infection got to the point where I thought a hot spear was being thrust slowly through my chest. And all this time, our savings were being used up. I tried to find out if I could get any sick benefits from an endowment policy I had. They said *no*. They didn't recognize CFIDS. I turned to the state, who said I did not qualify, and anyway, the amount they offered was so low as to be a joke. So, there we sat, piling up debt. Eventually we had to sell our home, which I found heartbreaking. Still, we are now in a quieter town, in a flat, and we have, by means of the sale, almost paid off all our debts. Small things make me very happy these days. All this time I was never diagnosed with CFIDS, or myalgic encephalomyelitis (ME), as it is known here. I often asked doctors and specialists, *Wasn't this "ME"? No*, they said, *there is no such thing*. Now the bad part of this was that I kept up false hopes of getting better. And after each infection left, I kept believing that this would be the time I got well. Only I never did. Even when there was no infection, and the weather or other cause wasn't giving me problems, and the depression was well under control, I found I was very, very weak. Most days I wouldn't even get dressed or shaved, but walked around inside our house in a bathrobe. I remember vividly walking to our P.O. box, which was about a kilometer away. I would often forget the key, but even when psychologically uplifting letters or packages arrived, I would stumble back home and literally fall into bed.

But going to the hospital was the worst. These were government, or state hospitals, and the deterioration they went through in the years between my running out of private medical assistance (to go to private hospitals with higher standards) and 1998 was, well, mind-blowing. I had heard of stories about various African countries going to pot, but much of this I hadn't believed. Well, I believe it now. Some brief pictures from these dreadful days: I recall waiting to see the doctor for a whole day, in the company of 400 or so other tired, sick people. I recall people fainting, and nurses just stepping over them. I remember people being told to go home because their medicines were not available today, and big men bursting out crying, unable to take the abuse any more. And I'll never forget the nurse who wouldn't allow me painkillers as this was "not her job." There was one case where I really lost my temper, and went and found my own file, contrary to hospital regulations. Somehow it was the waiting that was soul destroying. "Sit here, and wait." Then, two or three hours later, "move there" (and wait) and so on, often all day. I feel tired just remembering it.

In 1998, I was much better as regards getting infections. I only got four or five, one of which lasted three months. This is a great improvement. As for the future: I see all my big, grandiose dreams going up in smoke. I no longer plan, but rather, take small steps. I still nourish the hope that I can one day make a living as a writer, although the volume I can put out is relatively low.

So there you have it. The illness that isn't. It has caused a great deal of loss, both financially and emotionally, for something that isn't there. I am still tired, but trying to manage it well. I am eating a lot more vegetables, almost no sugar, trying to sleep regularly, taking adaptogens and vitamins. And I have to watch my activity. I could go on and on, but won't. What matters is that those hit by this "new illness" should receive help, both medical and social, so that they may carry on, rather than having to lose it all.

NOTE

1. "Chronic Disability Payments." Editorial. *The Wall Street Journal,* December 23, 1998, p. A14.

Chapter 21

Taking the Rap:
Parents, Blame, and Pediatric CFIDS

Mary Munson

Blame is as abundant as crabgrass in August. And like crabgrass, it spreads and fills the arid spaces where no solutions emerge. So it is no surprise that in the puzzling landscape of pediatric CFIDS, blame is rampant.

First, pediatric CFIDS seems the ultimate oxymoron. It cannot exist. Youth and exuberance are synonymous; we are worn out by the endless energy of children, their constant wiggling, running, jumping, so that "sit down" and "be quiet" are commands familiar to our collective unconscious. We have all heard them, indeed said them, a million times. So when a child becomes listless, with vague and persistent symptoms, we are alarmed. He must be brought "back to normal" as quickly as possible. Pediatricians usually provide potions and prescriptions (chill him down with ice) that work remarkably well. An army of gentle Mr. Rogerian soldiers, the pediatricians are accustomed to gratitude and adoration.

Well. CFIDS is a horse of a different color. A rare breed. An aberration. A nuisance, in fact. It has no apparent starting point (occasionally, it seems to) and certainly no obvious ending ("the fever has broken!"). It is chronic and stubborn, like thumb sucking or shyness, and like both of these, is thought to be probably caused by a default in the parental protocol. Rather than admit, "We have no cause, we have no cure, we have no clue (and maybe even we don't really care)," the medicine men more often lift a collective skeptical eyebrow and state: nothing is really sick here. Perhaps the parent is causing these symptoms. Or making them up. The search for causes and solutions is superseded by the search for where to assign the blame. The witch-hunt begins.

Mother's Day, 1999. I begin to write this article. It is for a book my daughter is editing—a book about CFIDS, the illness she herself has lived with for seven years. She is a talented writer and poet. I remember her birth very well; she was wide-eyed and watchful from the second of her birth. She was many things: exuberant, daring, yet also shy in some situations. She was my second daughter, following her sister by fourteen months. Like most mothers, I was full of hope, optimism, joy, and trepidation about this what-I-was-to-learn-quickly huge responsibility. I was an avid reader and so I read all I could about how to be a good mother. How to rear a healthy child. A smart child. A "well-adjusted" child. I think I was not unlike most young mothers.

I was therefore intrigued by the story of Mary O'Connor. Mary describes herself and her family as "ordinary" and "conventional." She would have preferred, I suppose, to remain ordinary, but instead she was thrust into an extraordinary drama, one she calls "One Family's Nightmare."[1] It began with Josie's flu. Josie, eleven years old, was on her way home from vacationing with her family when she started feeling sick: headache, muscle aches, nausea, sore throat.

I imagine myself as Josie's mother:

> I am worried. What is wrong? I hope that it will be over soon since caring for a sick child is quite boring for us both. I wonder whether to call the doctor. I hope I don't have to. Will the rest of us catch this?

After two weeks of the "flu," Josie started having other symptoms: difficulty sleeping, walking, and thinking; worsened headaches and nausea; sensitivity to light and sound.

My stream of consciousness again:

> Now I am getting alarmed. I am sure she is going to die. I am frantically trying to find some causes. I am calling my own mother, my friends who have children, too. What is wrong?

Here there is a long gap in Josie's story. Mary O'Connor picks up after Josie has been diagnosed with CFIDS for a *year* and her pediatrician had sent her to a neurologist for severe headaches.

Me:

> A year! Probably I felt relief at the diagnosis. It is not cancer! It is not terminal! Then puzzlement. What is it anyway? NEVER MIND. I can adapt to anything if only I can help my child. Thank you, God.

Then the adapting:

> School—she can't go; she is too weak.
>
> Her friends—she can't play; they lose interest.
>
> My friends—they are getting bored with an illness that won't go away; their eyes are glazing over; they stop asking about my daughter; they feel guilty about complaining that their own kids are "wearing them out"; they are secretly wondering: why on earth doesn't she *do* something?

Then the story of Mary O'Connor and her daughter Josie worsens. The neurologist, claiming that CFIDS is not a real illness, diagnoses the disease as Munchausen syndrome by proxy (MSBP). MSBP is a very weird name for a rare psychological illness in which a parent fakes or causes a child's symptoms in order to gain attention. Probably it was inevitable that this diagnosis would be attached at some point to parents of children with CFIDS.

In his prologue to the story of Mary O'Connor, Charles W. Lapp, MD, of Hunter-Hopkins Center in Charlotte, North Carolina, states that he is concerned with the increasing number of such cases. Too often, he says, physicians perceive the patient as "lazy" and the parents as "too lenient." Children faring poorly in school with many medical problems as well are sometimes considered to have MSBP, he relates. "Sadly, many physicians and social workers mistake the loving care of a concerned parent for neurosis and neglect; and many mistake chronic illness for a perverse illness career."[2]

Jane Colby, author of a book on pediatric CFIDS/ME in the United Kingdom titled *Zoe's Win,* collaborated with the health correspondent of the British Broadcasting Corporation (BBC) on a survey to determine the prevalence of these claims against families of ill children. The BBC later reported the statistics of their small sampling: the majority of families (59 percent) were told by doctors that their children's illness was psychological, 7 percent had been subjected to child protection proceedings (either threatened or carried out), and an astounding 4 percent had been labeled with Munchausen syndrome by proxy, 4,000 times the national rate of 1 in 100,000.[3]

This growing trend to tag the MSBP label on families of chronically ill children has spawned the organization MAMA, which stands for Mothers Against Munchausen Syndrome by Proxy Allegations. The Internet is the vehicle for linking families in what previously would have been solitary and overpowered protests. The conclusion to the case of Mary and Josie O'Connor is found there. Like Josie's illness itself, the story is lengthy. The good news is that Josie was allowed by the "authorities" to remain with her family. The bad news is that her illness continues and has worsened. The parents still risk losing custody if they are again accused of abusing her. The MSBP tattoo is a permanent one in their "past case history."

Another case of "blame the mum" syndrome was reported in the August 28, 1998, edition of *The Scotsman*. A twelve-year-old girl in East Lothian, Scotland, previously diagnosed with myalgic encephalomyelitis (as CFIDS is called in Great Britain), has been threatened with placement in foster care. Her local physician, Dr. Dayeel Goh, refused to accept the diagnosis of ME and referred the girl's case to government authorities because the mother would not consent to psychiatric treatment for her daughter. The curtain remains raised in this drama. An ME self-help group is assisting the mother in her case to be presented to the Children's Panel, the government authority who will decide whether this girl will remain in her mother's custody.[4]

One hundred thousand kids are estimated to have CFIDS. The layman understands it this way: If we find the cause, we can proceed to find the cure—that is the chronology. So the race is usually for the cause: of AIDS, of cancer, of CFIDS. The more mortality, the more legitimacy for the disease. In CFIDS, with its perplexing symptoms and indefinite outcome, both the cause and the cure have been frustratingly difficult to fathom. One asks why, though, in the case of CFIDS, is there then a conclusion that: (1) there is no disease, (2) the cause must be the individuals themselves and therefore under their control, or (3) it is a "psychological" ailment either dismissed or blamed on family pathology.

Manic-depressive disorder and stomach ulcers, for two, both once thought to be "psychosomatic," were given little medical attention until recent breakthrough discoveries in brain chemistry and viruses. CFIDS now lurks in that limbo of misunderstood illnesses. Pediatric CFIDS, less easily tied to stress as a cause, particularly lurks there. I notice no powerful righteous indignation as this blame is doled out. I notice the parents (here read "mother") sometimes willing to accept incriminations by authorities. Why is that? Here is my thesis:

The mother, source of everything, must be the source of this. She has beamed her way through those early years: What a pretty child! Thank you. You must be so proud! Yes, thank you. Secretly believing she is creating the perfect child, moving confidently, solving problems ("but how can I get him out of our bed?"), reading child psychology books, talking earnestly with other young mothers, feeling smug when those mothers are having problems ("he will not sit on the potty"), the mother is banking the credit for all that unfolds. There is a great divide—between the mothers and the childless. Certain commonalities among the mothers can never be truly understood by the childless. Another great divide exists between the ill and the well. Don't get sick and don't let your child get sick. The well own the world and merely tolerate the ill among them. The ill are marginalized.

So what a shocking surprise to find not only that one's child has become strangely ill but that the mother herself is seen as responsible for this illness! First comes the indignant anger: How dare they accuse me of fostering this illness, of coddling, of doing something to my child to make him want to become ill? To choose to become ill? Next comes the stepping back: What if they are right? Maybe I did cause it! Next comes the guilt: If they are right, I am a terrible person. Perhaps it is the innate knowledge that mothers have—that they can be responsible and held so for many trespasses against their own children—that makes them willing targets when a child becomes chronically ill. With the credit comes the blame.

Mother's Day, sometime later. I am finishing the piece. The huge outpouring of adoration on Mother's Day is in proportion—inverse proportion—to the bucketfuls of blame heaped on mothers the rest of the year. Everything from an offspring's sexual preferences to his or her annoying table manners can be accounted for by shining the spotlight on the mother. So Mary O'Connor and the other mothers were probably not overly surprised at the attitudes of physicians, social workers, teachers, and friends. They were probably astounded, however, to find a charge of child abuse leveled against them.

The real losers in this blame game are the children. With parents (specifically mothers) willing to tolerate accusations against them, perhaps seeing no other alternative, and with their critics willing to level charges of blame, the focus shifts away from the arduous and tedious work of making children well again. Let's get on with it.

NOTES

1. O'Connor, Mary. "One Family's Nightmare." (Posted at the Web site for Mothers Against Munchausen Syndrome by Proxy Allegations (MAMA) <www.msbp.com/maryo.htm>. MAMA address: 1407 Ranch Drive, Senatobia, MS 38668.)

2. Lapp, Charles. "A CFS Tragedy." (Posted at the Web site for MAMA.)

3. Colby, Jane. *Zoe's Win.* Ongar, UK: Dome Vision, 2000, p. 72.

4. Breen, Stephen. "Doctors in bitter row over case of ME girl." *The Scotsman.* August 28, 1998, p. 5 (last edition).

PART V:
FATE AND FAITH

Chapter 22

Kismet

Floyd Skloot

My brother Philip was buried on the morning of my fiftieth birthday. Earlier that week, he had decided to stop dialysis treatments, so his death was not really a surprise.

But it was a shock. My sister-in-law called just after dawn and I snatched up the phone, turning on my knees, naked, to lean over the bed as though in prayer. Elaine said hello, then issued a sound I did not at first recognize. The phone in our bedroom is an ancient, staticky cordless with a replacement universal antenna that falls off whenever I pick up the unit, so I assumed that the sound was just her voice breaking up over the thousand miles between us.

But my wife, Beverly, knew at once what she heard coming through the unit and the bones of my skull. She bounded out of bed, ran into the next room, picked up the phone in there and began comforting Elaine before I could let the truth seep in.

We had last seen Philip two months earlier. During that visit, for the first time, he had begun to speak about dying. On Friday night, he interrupted a dinner-table discussion of the virtues of root vegetables to say he thought he had about six months left. Provided he continued receiving dialysis four times a week. *I'm okay with this. I've had a good life.* He gestured toward Elaine and his left hand landed on top of his buttered bread, which made him chuckle, then shrug, then eat the chocolate chip cookie he had been hiding in his right hand.

Near the end, when he weighed 264 pounds, my brother was a vestige of his former self. He sat quietly in his recliner or wheelchair, listening, a mellow smile on his face, gray hair flattened in back and spread like a fan above his ears. When he spoke his voice was deeper and slower than it had ever been, tamped down. What he had to say was offered in counterpoint, as a comment on what he heard rather than as part of the main melody.

Philip was fifty-seven. In his apartment, he liked to strip right down to basics, white boxer shorts and V-neck T-shirt, or maybe a pair of loose sweatpants while the air conditioning blasted. Without the black wraparound shades, he kept his sightless eyes closed. Without the false teeth, he kept his mouth shut but loved to work his gums sideways across each other. His skin, stippled with odd growths, bore the soft ocher shade of renal failure and stung whenever he was touched. There was a hump at the base of his neck. He could barely walk, soles numbed, muscles atrophied, balance in shambles. He needed help to stand and could not get himself up off the toilet or take a shower by himself. He had trouble breathing and when he slept, slumped in the recliner, his face erupted in tics.

He looked exactly like our grandmother Kate in the months before she died in 1965. She was then seventy-nine.

In his heyday my brother weighed 375 pounds but moved with uncanny grace, as though the planet held him in place with a different kind of force than the rest of us. He was a successful gambler, a savvy player of games, an unlikely ladies' man. He knew odds; he counted cards. Over the years, he sold pressure-sensitive papers or envelopes or shoes or metals, always expanding his territory, on the go. When he could no longer walk well or see well enough to drive, he sold computer hardware by phone, what he disdainfully called inside sales. He was the kind of guy you instinctively trust, a sell-sand-to-the-Saudis type, and his word was good. He was the joke-a-minute sort, the life of the party, suavely smiling, cigarette cupped in his palm, wise to the ways of the world. Even blind, he would give his wife directions when they drove together through the streets of San Francisco, saying "turn left here," or "bear right at that Texaco station." He knew what he knew. He loved the spotlight, the lead, and he was never very interested in blending into the background.

For casual wear, my brother favored brightly colored shirts and contrasting golf slacks. He claimed visual space, flaunting his size, proclaiming that he had nothing to hide. I have a photograph of Philip posed beside his tall, slender wife before a fancy evening out; he is wearing a red sports jacket with fuschia accents, a fuschia tie and red shoes to go with the white shirt and red-and-white checked slacks. As always, the thick black hair is carefully pompadoured.

To eat with him was to witness pleasure carried to the level of torture. Restaurant owners and chefs fawned over him, the maître d'hôtel and maître de cuisine lavishing attention on his vast table of friends, waitresses bringing free desserts and aperitifs. He tipped everyone twice. I remember eating a five-course dinner with him one Saturday night at an Italian restaurant in New York's East Village, Mario's, then stopping for doughnuts on the short drive to his home in New Jersey, then watching him eat a sandwich before going to bed. My sleep that night was one endless nightmare. Early next morning, there was a full table of traditional Jewish Sunday brunch foods, bagels and nova with cream cheese, smoked sable and sturgeon, whitefish chubs, lox wings, ruggelach.

Afterward, we drove to the batting range and swatted line drives in the blistering August heat. I weighed less than half of what he weighed, but felt rotund as Babe Ruth and was not sure I could manage a swing without my arms thumping my belly.

Our grandfather Philip, my brother's namesake, was born in the old country in the fall of 1880. The old country was Russia or Poland or Lithuania, depending on the year in question, though in the late nineteenth century it was part of the Russian empire designated as The Pale of Settlement by Tsar Alexander III, the only place where Jews were legally authorized to settle. Skluts came from Volozhin, between Minsk and Vilnius, in what was known as White Russia and is now part of Belarus.

It was and remains a small town. But its renowned Jewish academy or yeshiva was known throughout the Jewish world, a place that was led by such great rabbis as Rav Chaim or Rav Joseph Baer Soloveichik and that attracted Talmudic scholars. The Hebrew poet Hayyim Nahman Bialik and essayist/fiction writer Micah Joseph Berdichevsky studied there.

As Paul Johnson notes in his book *A History of the Jews,* "in the last half-century of imperial Russia, the official Jewish regulations formed an enormous monument to human cruelty." It was a preview for Nazi policy. To be a Jew in Volozhin was to be constantly at risk from Poles, Cossacks, Catholics, Tsarist loyalists, Nazis, and to survive required both vigilance and resilience.

Beset by violence, transformed by invasion the way a cell is transformed by a virus, Volozhin's destiny was to be always under attack. Like a human body perpetually challenged by pathogens, the community's collective defense mechanisms became rewired, organized to be continually on alert. We became a people focused on self-defense, locked into patterns of resistance, guarded even when there was no threat.

Prayer, communal solidarity, the development of niche skills, bribery, conversion—these were typical external forms of coping. In *A Promised Land,* Mary Antin's classic 1912 memoir of East European Jewish life and immigration, a sense of resignation underlies Jewish creativity in the face of continued calamity: "But what can one do? The people said, with a shrug of the shoulders that expresses the helplessness of the Pale. What can one do? One must live."

At constant risk, people either adapted or perished. Current theories about evolutionary biology suggest that there would have been internal forms of coping as well, biological adaptations to prolonged stress that mirrored the external adaptations, ultimately weakening the body as they preserved it, overburdening the immune system. In time, a pattern of neurologically mediated behavior evolved that closed off responses irrelevant to self-protection. In a sense, my brother and I came from people whose biological adaptation to stress had a self-destructive component. Programmed to biologically circle the wagons, our immunological responses were maladaptive—we eat ourselves up with worry. This was the secret baggage brought to America from the old country, and whether or not the theory is correct, the metaphorical implications are compelling.

After increasingly anti-Semitic restrictions imposed by Alexander III, and an escalation of pogroms, four Sklut brothers left Volozhin in 1892. Two settled in South Africa, where the family name became Sloot; two, named Eliahu and Samuel, came to New York, where they were processed at Ellis Island as Skloot.

Grandfather Philip, a scholarly former student prepared to enroll at the Volozhin yeshiva, a reader of books and nascent arguer of interpretive points, went to work in an undershirt factory. Shortly afterward, his father—our great-grandfather Eliahu—died of a heart attack. Eliahu was in his mid-fifties when he died. He never got to see his younger son save enough money to own his own grocery store, or marry an émigré from Bialystok named Kate Tatarsky and open his own live kosher poultry market.

Like Eliahu, grandfather Philip's life was short and his end sudden. A diabetic, he died of a heart attack in his eldest daughter's arms in 1939. He was fifty-nine. And like the two generations before him, our own father's life, also etched with diabetes, ended by heart attack. He was fifty-three.

It is easy to look at this pattern and conclude that our destiny is to die young of heart disease and the complications of diabetes. It is fate, kismet. The three generations of fathers we know about all did so. Whether due to evolutionary biology's maladaptive changes or to long-standing genetic tendencies, we are genetic patsies and there is not much we can do.

In essence, this was my brother's view. He ate wildly, almost contemptuously, in the face of his inheritance. He smoked to the same rhythm, often four packs of cigarettes a day. Aggressively sedentary, he was an accomplished napper, a spectator and kibitzer of fine style and volume. He was resigned to the inevitability of early death and chose to live high while he lived. In a sense, he converted; he joined the enemy.

My own view was the exact opposite. I dieted fanatically, buying ever more sensitive bathroom scales and kitchen scales, measuring and apportioning nearly everything I took in, keeping elaborate diaries of my running with details added of sleep and weight and estimated calories burned. Never smoked, logged nearly 2,500 miles of running a year, ate all the miracle foods from oat bran to salmon to Egg Beaters omelettes, and took all the supplements. I worried and wrote poems about dying young, and had a will drawn up before I had anything of value to leave behind. I also thought I was managing stress, having developed all those outlets for it, but of course was so intense about this that it made my brother laugh. Then, in 1988, my health collapsed utterly. During a long airplane flight, I was exposed to a virus that targeted my brain, scarring it with lesions that remain today, and my already-compromised immune system misread all the signs, going into permanent overdrive. I remain, nine years later, totally disabled, neurologically impaired and confined, for the most part, to home.

There was something romantic about the assumption of being marked for an early end. Like Mickey Mantle, our hero when we were growing up, or like settlers beyond The Pale who hear Cossacks in every shift of the wind, my brother and I felt shadowed by mortality. Philip, adopting the Mantle method, went for broke, living it up in the terms that made most sense to him; I became something of a genetic ascetic, denying nearly everything that my brother emphasized. He was a hellion and I was a good boy. We were, as ever, quite a team.

But the truth of the matter is that genetic tendencies toward diabetes, heart disease, and obesity, however evolved, are not necessarily death sentences. The geneticist Steve Jones writes, in *The Language of Genes,* that "a harmful gene can sometimes become obvious only when the environment changes." Both Philip and I have a genetic predisposition to diabetes, but it is not a genetic sentence to the disease unless we create the right environment for the harmful gene to flourish.

According to *The Merck Manual,* 80 to 90 percent of the people with type II diabetes mellitus, the common adult-onset, non-insulin-dependent form of the disease which my brother developed, are obese. In these cases, the body still produces insulin—the hormone responsible for absorption of glucose into cells for energy production—but in insufficient amounts to meet the body's needs, especially when the body is overweight. Not only is it possible to prevent, or at least to delay, the onset of diabetes, but the disease can be controlled through careful management of diet, exercise, and the use of drugs. My brother did none of these things, either before or after diabetes began to change his life.

I remember visiting Philip in Fremont, California, in 1984. He took me on a sightseeing tour of the area, driving up into the hills of Alameda County and the Sunoi Regional Wilderness, weaving all over the road in his struggle with fading eyesight. After dinner at his favorite restaurant, which included a double order of zabaglione—a beaten egg yolk, sugar, and liqueur concoction—for dessert, he insisted on driving home. Suddenly, he pulled onto the shoulder of the highway, sighed, and just made it over to the passenger seat before falling into a sleep that approached coma.

In 1991, Philip flew up to visit me in Portland, Oregon. He was the last to emerge from the plane, and I was glad he could not see my reaction. He was gray-haired and his teeth, which had steadily begun to spread into gaps, were now a gleaming row of ill-fitting chompers that distorted his mouth. His eyeglasses were thick and sturdy as mugs, with a special insert in the right lens for magnification. Only his right eye had vision, but he obviously could not see well enough to walk with confidence and held his arms poised in front of his chest like a wrestler. He was hungry after the flight and wanted to stop for a sweet roll before we left the airport.

The last meal we ate together in a restaurant, in early spring of 1997, culminated in Philip's ordering baked Alaska. He had not liked his appetizer of raw clams, nor his shrimp cocktail, and had not been able to finish his salmon. Wheelchair tucked under the table's edge, he signaled for the waitress all throughout the meal, wanting dessert before our entrées had arrived, lost in time, and unaware that we had been seated for just twenty minutes. He could not get enough water, though he was not supposed to drink much in the days between dialysis. He was edgy, unable to listen to conversation, and his usual smile was gone. I knew that we were seeing the end of Philip's journey, when even a fine meal could no longer please him. Only when his dessert arrived did he settle down, and when it was done he smiled in turn at each of us.

One Monday evening in the fall of 1958, my brother announced that he wanted to audition for a local theater production of *Kismet* on Thursday. "What else am I going to do?" he asked.

He figured he would play Hajj the poet-beggar and get to sing "Fate!" in his rich baritone. *What fate, what fate is mine?* Hajj had easy songs to put over on an audience, Philip thought, songs that took acting talent rather than operatic pipes. It would be a cinch. Or maybe he would play the Caliph, lighten up the voice a little so he could be the beau and croon the great love songs like "Stranger in Paradise."

We had moved from Brooklyn to Long Island the year before, following his high school graduation, and Philip knew no one in the town where we lived. Stranded, he said, just like Hajj. So it would be method acting. Being in the play might be a good way to make friends, to meet girls. Especially girls, since he was spending all his free time now driving to and from Brooklyn for dates and was too tired to get up for work in the mornings.

At nineteen, he was finished with his half-hearted attempt at college, where playing intramural football had gradually become his major. Employed in the Manhattan garment district, he was learning the children's dress business from our mother's Uncle Sam, who owned Youngland. He wanted to sell, but had to begin by sweeping floors. He hated it. He would drive into the city from our new Long Island home every morning at 7:00, leaving a half-hour after our father, who worked only a few blocks from Youngland. They would arrive back home in their separate cars at nearly the same time, ravenous for dinner, but would never commute together, for reasons they seemed to agree upon without ever having to talk about them. After dinner, there was nothing for him to do but sit around the house and bicker with our parents or play endless games of Careers with me. He hated that too.

I was eleven and my job for Wednesday afternoon was to prepare Philip's audition song for him. He was not supposed to sing any-thing from *Kismet* and had chosen Tennessee Ernie Ford's hit from three years earlier, "Sixteen Tons." I had to listen to the record and write down the lyrics. And they had better be perfect, even if I had to listen to it a thousand and one times. *Some people say a man is made out of mud. A poor man's made out of muscle and blood.*

"What's this?" he asked on Wednesday night, when I handed him the page of lyrics. Certain lines had a heavy X in the margin.

"Snaps. You have to snap your fingers there when you sing."

He shook his head. "I'll do the snapless version. You never see an Arab snap his fingers when he sings."

Kismet, which opened on Broadway in December 1953, has an unusual pedigree. Basing a musical's book on an existing novel or play was a Broadway tradition—the Gershwins did it with *Porgy and Bess;* Rodgers and Hammerstein did it with *Carousel* and *South Pacific.* The script of *Kismet* is based upon a popular World War I-era play by Edward Knoblock, set in Baghdad, that used the grandeur of the Arabian Nights as background for a romance between a beggar's daughter and a noble caliph despite the machinations of the Wazir. But unlike the great musicals of the period, the score of *Kismet* was completely unoriginal. Its music actually came from mid-nineteenth-century Russia, composed there by a chemist and professor of medicine named Aleksandr Borodin. Its lyrics, however, were written nearly a century later by two Americans, Robert Wright and George Forrest, who made a theatrical career out of putting words to the melodies of dead composers. They had already turned Edvard Grieg's music into *The Song of Norway,* Sergei Rachmaninoff's into *Arya,* and Victor Herbert's into *Gypsy Lady,* so their formula was well tested. For *Kismet,* they applied lyrics to Borodin's *Polovtsian Dances* for "Stranger in Paradise," "He's in Love" and "Not Since Ninevah." They used a love duet from the opera *Prince Igor* for "The Olive Tree" and another melody from earlier in that opera to create "Rhymes Have I." The Notturno of Borodin's String Quartet no. 2 in D Major was used for "And This Is My Beloved" and a theme from elsewhere in the quartet gave them "Was I Wazir?". Symphony no. 1 yielded "Gesticulate," Symphony no. 2 produced "Fate," and *In the Steppes of Central Asia* turned into "Sands of Time." Listening to a recording of Borodin is like listening to Wright and Forrest's Overture. At a Portland Chamber Orchestra performance of the D Major Quartet, I drew angry stares for singing along with the Notturno.

Clearly, *Kismet* is a classic of adaptation. Taking the genetic code of Borodin's music, grafting it onto an ancient Middle Eastern fable and writing fresh lyrics, Wright and Forrest did something wholly new with what they were given. They created an alternative destiny, a new life out of Borodin's material, giving it quintessentially American features. Fittingly, the winner of Broadway's Tony Award in 1953 for excellence in musical composition was Aleksandr Borodin, who had died in 1887.

Philip's audition for *Kismet* was a success in the sense that he got a part in the production. But he was cast as the Wazir and had only one song to sing. He would be going to rehearsals every night for two months in order to sing one song! I knew he would hate that and thought it was my fault.

But I was wrong. He reveled in the cruelty of the character, the wicked minister of state who dismembered suspects arm by arm and ear by ear and joint by joint, who sealed an embezzling tax collector in a pot of glue and hung 700 men "by their fuzz" in a prison pen. *Was I Wazir? I was!* Philip played the Wazir as a Cossack, modeling the role on those stories we had grown up with, tales of vicious torturers who preyed on Jews. I read him his cues in our living room and saw how hard he worked. Eyes bulging and fists clenched like our mother's when she was angry, voice going flat like our father's when he was about to erupt, he used everything he knew. In performance, he was riveting; with his sinister and musical laugh, his relish in delivering the song, even in his death by drowning, he stole the show. *I hacked and hatcheted and cleft until no one but me is left!*

Kismet has an underlying motif of sensory confusion, of difficulty in figuring out how to read the signs. *Fate,* Hajj sings, *can be the trap in your path.* It can *weave the evil and good in one design. Is it good? Is it ill? Am I blessed, am I cursed? Is it honey on my tongue or brine? What fate what fate is mine?*

I cannot listen to the soundtrack without chills. It speaks to something so deep within me, a mix of fraternal memories and fears and pride that seem never to have released their hold. I also hear in the exotic music and back story a theme that has dominated our lives: the mysteries of fate, of kismet, as played out in the blood. My brother and I share a legacy of bad genes and confusion over what to do about them.

I have never forgotten a childhood dream about my brother. It probably occurred in 1954, when I was six, since I woke up in the room we shared in our Brooklyn apartment. I got out of bed and went across the room to his, carefully leaning over his body to determine whether he was still there and still alive.

The dream was set in that room, which was four stories up above the building's enclosed courtyard and looked down a brick alcove onto the space where we played stickball. My brother, glasses off, dressed in an undershirt and pajama pants, was clinging to the window ledge. He was calling to me. I tried to get out of bed, but the covers were too heavy. Just as he lost his grip, I managed to squirm free and run to the window. But the air was thick, like the ocean at Long Beach where we went on hot spring afternoons, and I could not move fast enough. He began to drift away, floating like a feather rather than plummeting to the courtyard. His right hand still reached for me; his eyes were fixed on mine. He was silent, all his hopes grappled to my outstretched arms that could do nothing for him.

Beverly and I began visiting Philip regularly in 1995. Every three months, we would fly to San Jose on a Thursday afternoon and stay until early Monday morning. It was the end game. We all knew that, but since he never spoke about being terminally ill, we only discussed such matters out of his hearing.

At first, he would be sitting in his wheelchair at the gate to greet us, duded up in shades and windbreaker, head tilted back to hear what Elaine whispered as she bent over the chair's back with her hands on the grips. He loved to hug Beverly, this tall and willowy blonde sister-in-law of his that he had never actually seen but clearly approved of. We would head for the baggage claim together, me with my cane and Philip being pushed in his chair, and he would lay out the weekend's plans for where we eat each night.

A rhythm developed through the next two years. Thursday evening we would dine at a vegetarian restaurant in San Jose, in honor of Beverly's preferences, and Philip would joke about his passion for bok choy. I had never known him to compromise when it came to food, but he was elegant in his consideration now. On Friday we would drive him to dialysis in the morning, dropping him off at 9:00 and returning at 1:00. Then we would bring him home, keep him company as he ate a sandwich and napped until the cooking programs came on television at 4:00. We prepared dinner on Fridays, since Elaine worked all day. Saturdays were for rest and then dinner at fancy restaurants in San Francisco; Sundays were for dinner with their two grown children.

Gradually, time fell apart. Philip was no longer able to meet us at the gate, waiting instead in the car while we got our baggage. We began eating in restaurants closer to their apartment on Thursdays and then, by mid-1997, went straight home and ordered takeout dinners. Friday, his stays at the dialysis center got shorter, until at last he was there for less than an hour, gradually diminishing his treatments and growing ever sicker as the toxins normally removed by dialysis built up. After being hooked to the machine through an indwelling catheter directly above his heart, Philip would doze for a few minutes. Awake, he could not remember how long ago he had arrived, but believed that he had to get home immediately. Neither the attendants nor the nurses nor the doctors nor I could convince him that he had only been there a half hour. He slept for six hours afterward instead of three and could not eat the dinners we prepared. On Saturdays, he could not venture out for the trips to Monterey or to San Francisco, as before, and on Sundays he could barely stay awake during the family visits. He talked less and less.

Then over dinner the last Friday we saw him, Philip spoke about being okay with death, about having a good life, and stuck his hand in the buttered bread. He was surrounded by pill bottles and the apparatus for injecting himself in the abdomen with insulin. He was surrounded by cookies. He was surrounded by family and love. He was surrounded.

One morning in September 1997, about two months after my brother died, I was sitting on the living room couch listening to music. It was just after breakfast. Across the room was the collage of photographs I had assembled on the weekend he died. One showed my brother, age eight, holding me in his arms shortly after I was born. He is dressed in an undershirt and striped pajama pants, sitting on the edge of his bed, and has unwrapped me like a gift. My discarded blankets lie next to him. Not quite smiling, hunched there in a room crowded by the crib crammed against the wall behind him, Philip looks confused but resigned. *Am I blessed? Am I cursed?* In a second photograph, I stand between him and our cousin Phyllis, both squatting before a parking lot fence through which the rear ends of late-1940s Oldsmobiles and Chevrolets can be seen. Philip is displaying a white windup toy dog to the camera, obviously something just given to me, and Phyllis holds a plastic dog bone. They are both smiling and I have the same resigned, confused look on my two-year-old's face that Philip had in the earlier photo. The final image was taken a half year ago, after our last restaurant meal with Philip. He is at the head of the table, his wife beside him with her hand clasped in his, and a single red tulip juts from its vase, tilted toward them as though drawn to their warmth. I am next to Elaine, looking across the table at my wife. We are all smiling. We seem almost giddy at being together. There is nothing held back and there are no questions in the air. His expression says *I've had a good life.*

As the sun rose just high enough above the oaks to shine into our windows, the Notturno from Aleksandr Borodin's D Major Quartet began. Its exquisite, tender theme—the movement essentially has only one theme, repeated and varied among the strings for eight minutes —was announced by the cello and floated across the air. For the first time since my brother died, I began to cry and could not stop until the music ended.

My brother had been dying for so long that I had time to prepare myself. As his physical presence dwindled, memories of him loomed everywhere. The transition to holding on to him as pure memory was relatively simple. But somewhere along the way, I had skipped a step, held my grief in and instead built a shrine to my brother's dogged destiny.

Now I see it all tinged with regret, even anger, because his death was unnecessary. Through the years of excess, he could be provoked to fury by any suggestion that he temper his behavior; at the end, he acknowledged his mistakes and worried about the fate of his son, whose habits are a direct copy of Philip's. The riddle of *Kismet* remained unsolved for my brother. The honey on his tongue was in fact brine and what he construed as good was ill. He sought to embrace in life the very things that would kill him. That, rather than the more mundane genetic inheritance or the facts of renal failure, is the real end of the story.

Chapter 23

Spiritual Healing, Holistic Healing, and the White Light Fascists

Caitlin MacEwan

I have worked for twenty-one of my thirty-five years with alternative healing methods. I started so early because I've had CFIDS-type symptoms for much of my life and as I got older the symptoms worsened. My mother sought out alternative methods for me at first; then I studied these methods and employed them myself. I have spent many years in therapy, support groups, and spiritual healing circles. I have studied psychic and energetic healing. And I have led ongoing groups in spiritual practice and energy work. At my worst, completely bedridden for years and convinced I was dying, I was so seriously ill, so deeply fatigued on every level of my being, that despite knowing and having taught these spiritual healing methods, I was completely unable to muster my will or vital energy to use them. You can't meditate when your brain isn't functioning. And it's very, very hard to have spiritual focus when your body is in agony. It didn't matter how much I believed in the power of my will to change my energy and my body. I had run on a combination of adrenaline, caffeine, and willpower for so many years that there was simply no reserve left within me. For awhile I didn't even seek medical help. I believed that if I couldn't heal myself by my own power, it simply couldn't be done. It sounds horribly arrogant to me, now, but some of my past experiences had led me to think this way.

I was trained in a spiritual tradition that has a strong belief in magic. I've seen incredible physical changes happen in response to

---

"Spiritual Healing, Holistic Healing, and White Light Fascists" is excerpted from a much longer and more personal essay of the same title.

metaphysical methods. Though we all like to believe that our intelligence and insight can protect us from exploitation, sometimes physical and emotional pain can make us ignore our warning bells and fall into stupid and dangerous situations. I was particularly vulnerable to exploitation in the early years of my battle with CFIDS, as I had seemingly willed myself into significant periods of remission over the years. And earlier in my life I had confounded the doctors by healing from a back injury that they said would paralyze me. I thought I was invincible.

When the New Age boom of the 1980s hit my community, I was open-minded. What I severely underestimated was my own level of need and gullibility, and how this could play into the hands of "spiritual" con artists. In the desperate early years of my illness, I had some awful run-ins with the "you create your own reality" New Age followers. Prompted by friends, I took a series of expensive training seminars to learn a technique of healing based upon breath work, forgiveness, and attitudinal changes. Allegedly, we would resolve any trauma and blocked energy that we were still carrying around, unconsciously, from the experience of birth; and we would learn to have more loving relationships, thereby healing our lives in the process.

I was instructed that if I wrote hundreds of affirmations, I would get well. If this didn't cure my illness, well, it meant that I just didn't love myself enough and that I needed to "do more breath work" and "write more affirmations" and "do more trainings and seminars" (these are actual quotes, by the way). I was also encouraged to give up my friends who weren't involved in this group, which, thankfully, I didn't do.

In the mid-1980s, the "White Light" infection was epidemic. One of my health care practitioners at this time, a chiropractor, became caught in this trend and actually told me that the reason my immune system was failing was because I simply didn't want to be well. Or, I just didn't want it badly enough. I left her office in tears and never went back.

Such blame-the-victim attitudes seriously distract people from looking for the real causes of their illness. Ironically, it's exactly the sort of people who want to delve deep—to find the core reasons for their problems—who are drawn to New Age groups. Although therapy and support groups can help people with CFIDS (PWCs) resolve emotional issues and adapt to the limitations imposed by their illness, that's not what these groups do. With their quick-fix, pop-psychology seminars and "support groups" run for financial gain, they deny the reality of most illness, believing it is all in the mind.

Most of the people involved in this fad of the privileged (or sometimes, and even sadder, those without privilege but who desperately need help) actively discourage any sort of political, economic, or social analysis of the conditions that cause pain and illness in our culture. They see all problems as personal, the self as center of the universe. While I knew that homophobia, racism, misogyny, poverty, and war aren't caused by the individuals experiencing oppression, the people around me were subtly and not-so-subtly implying that they were.

During my brief involvement with this group of New Agers, I heard people blamed for all conceivable sorts of tragedies. I once stood and cheered as an elderly Jewish man stood up and confronted a very well-known New Age author and seminar leader, demanding that she explain the "wonderful growth experience" of the Holocaust, and whether, in her opinion, the Jews had caused the experience. It was one of the best moments in that whole morass, this man shaking with righteous anger, refusing to be ignored.

Though the spiritual community I later joined was, for the most part, more grounded, political, and realistic, I would still sometimes meet fellow spiritual practitioners who seemed to be intelligent and perceptive, only to have them react to my physical limitations with the same old blaming clichés. Or, alternately, people would refuse to believe I was really sick, precisely because I *am* spiritual, and back then I was still capable of appearing healthy for short periods of time. Appallingly enough, sometimes the same people would blame me and then claim I wasn't really sick. Oh, and lest I forget the real gem: "What a wonderful opportunity for growth and learning!" I got to the point where I was ready to wish the same "opportunity" right onto them. These morons also thought anger was always "bad" and would never hesitate to tell me how spiritually stunted I must be if any kind of injustice angered me. What I really saw in them was a fear of all strong emotions, a fear of the truth, and a desperate fear of admitting their own limitations.

What I have come to value is the true healing and compassion that is found in radical honesty, depth, and vulnerability. It's the antithesis of what these New Age gurus were preaching. If their philosophy were right, there would be no disease in the world, no poverty, no oppression, no death. Most New Age "positive thinking" is just Christian Science-derived denial dressed up in more exotic, and modern, clothing. It's sexy because they claim they can heal our deepest pain. It sounds too good to be true, and it is. I had been far away from the White Light Fascists for years before I wound up completely bedridden and deathly ill, but, oddly, I didn't connect my shame and my reluctance to try "chemical" drugs with these experiences.

Two of the main things that enabled me to break free from the inertia of self-blame and mobilize my spiritual energies for healing were SSRIs (selective serotonin reuptake inhibitors) for my depression and severe insomnia, and a drug to inhibit the growth of a benign pituitary tumor that was severely disrupting my hormonal levels. But I resisted these "unnatural" treatments for years, due to my holistic background. Apparently, the tumor had been there for years, unsuspected. It had been causing some of the symptoms that I had assumed to be psychological and had therefore blamed upon myself. The usual response to this sort of tumor is surgery to remove it, but due to the CFIDS I'm not a good candidate for surgery. Like a good little spiritual girl, I used the visualization method on it for years before I finally broke down and tried the drugs.

I want to stress that depression and CFIDS are not the same thing. Treating the depression did not cure my fevers, flulike chills and body aches, infections, headaches, joint pain, sore throats, and severe fatigue. What it did was help me to cope, improve my quality of life, and keep me from giving up. It enabled my brain to function again so I could resume my spiritual practice. I'm very lucky that the drugs helped me, as the pain of CFIDS, the nightmare of insomnia, and the frequently severe secondary depression have driven numerous people with CFIDS to suicide.

Many people in the holistic communities—usually those who have never dealt with serious illness themselves—are adamant in trying to convince PWCs that "natural" is always better than "chemical." The Internet, in particular, is full of self-styled "healers" dispensing this advice. Lately this has taken the form of recommending one or two popular herbs to replace drugs, and shaming the PWC if and when the herbs don't help, or don't help sufficiently. Usually these herbal recommendations are passed on by people with little to no training or experience in herbalism. I grow and use herbs extensively and rely on them as part of my health care program. But, like drugs, many herbs can be toxic, harmful, or ineffective if prepared incorrectly, used in the wrong situation, or taken in inappropriate amounts or for too long (or short) a time. Herbs are not a cure-all.

Quack "healers" thrive wherever there is chronic illness. They profit on despair and brainwash the ill into even deeper despair. While a great deal of good may be found in a number of alternative healing modalities, the unregulated nature of some of these practices can provide a haven for predators. Those with mild illness can often recover quite well using only "natural" methods. For instance, in the early years of my illness I had significant remissions from (only) Chinese herbs and acupuncture. But those of us who are more severely disabled can reach a point where we also need to use prescription drugs. There's nothing wrong with this, and we deserve to not be shamed about it. It is shaming and negative to guilt-trip people in the guise of unasked-for "spiritual advice"; and following it up with "I love you unconditionally" doesn't mitigate it, it only hides the speaker behind a veil of self-righteousness.

The worst period of sickness for me was when I let a New Age quack talk me into stopping my "more invasive" allopathic treatments —all drugs, and even megavitamins, blood products, and herbs that were used in a concentrated, injectable form. I backslid severely and it took me years to recover.

A particularly horrible insult I have seen directed at PWCs by at least one self-proclaimed "spiritual" healer is the accusation that PWCs are looking for an identity and somehow find it in identifying as PWCs. What this appallingly ignorant accusation ignores is that CFIDS isn't an identity but a medical diagnosis. It's an illness, not a chosen lifestyle. What a hateful assumption—that someone would want to be stricken with this pain and struggle. This also ignores the evidence that most of us PWCs were extremely high-functioning overachievers before becoming completely disabled. I pushed through my symptoms for years. I'd show up at an event and appear to be energetic and strong. But what few people knew was that, despite my sometimes-impressive performance, even in demanding leadership roles, I was pushing myself through almost-crippling pain and fever. And then I would go home and collapse completely from opportunistic infections, severe bronchitis, flu, strep throat, and/or adrenal exhaustion for days, or weeks, at a time before becoming physically functional enough to start the cycle again. Then the necessary recovery time would take months. Now it's been years. It's quite probable that the severity of my illness is partially due to my ongoing refusal, especially in the beginning, to rest and accept my physical limitations.

I still struggle with my own denial. It's too painful to always remember how limited I am by this disease. My denial not only kept me from getting proper medical treatment, it kept me from looking after my own, and my family's, financial needs. I was too sick to work, even part time, for years before I finally applied for disability benefits. As sick as I was, every day I would assume that this was just temporary, and that the next day I'd be better and soon I'd be perfectly healthy. It was too painful for me to entertain any other possibility. Getting disability payments meant facing up to the possibility that I wasn't going to get better in the foreseeable future, and my mind simply couldn't encompass that.

People do have "miracle" remissions from severe illnesses such as cancer and multiple sclerosis, and sometimes they attribute this to "positive thinking." But in my considerable experience, these cases are the exception, and seem to be just as likely to happen to people who go out dancing as to people who take their herbs and meditate. The crime is when people misrepresent these few exceptions as the rule. They also don't seem to realize, or care, that CFIDS is a very different disease than, say, cancer. We're still in the very beginning stages of figuring out what does and doesn't work with this disease.

When I first began speaking up about the limitations of spiritual healing (something of a heretical act in some of the circles I've run in), some people perceived me as putting down "natural" remedies and/or implying that spiritual healing never happens. Perhaps I was overcompensating in my criticism, due to the crazy extents I'd seen some people go to with their magical thinking. The truth is, I'm about as alternative as you can get in most ways. But my understanding of alternative healing methods may be based on a completely different series of experiences, scholarship, and research than someone else with, say, a more yuppie New Age perspective, or someone who doesn't really have experience with the natural remedies they so blithely champion. I was just saying that "natural" isn't always better, safer, or effective.

Although I do respect and honor our rights to our different opinions, twenty-odd years in the spiritual healing communities have shown me that many people who adopt the "you create your own reality" credo go through distinct stages with it. For a period of months or years they're enthusiastic converts. They alienate people with their platitudes, delusions, and grandiosity, then they rationalize this alienation by blaming others for not being "evolved" enough or "positive" enough to understand them. Then, eventually, something profound and healing happens—the goddesses bless them with tragedy. They see loved ones, or themselves, some of the most spiritually evolved people they know, go through horrible suffering. Life happens. And slowly they realize that we are all only cocreators of our reality—we are not the center of the universe. Each one of us is only one bright spirit spark among all the others, and all of these factors, from the spirits down to the microbes, are creating this dance together. None of us is above this dance. None of us is below it. We are all just part of it.

Chapter 24

CFIDS, Suffering, and the Divine

James Rotholz

The points of intersection between anthropology and theology are rather obscure for most people. Anthropology, in its essence, attempts to understand and see life through the eyes of the person or group being studied—the other. Theology, on the other hand, tries to provide a divine or spiritually informed point of view. Strangely enough, it was chronic fatigue immune dysfunction syndrome (CFIDS) that brought the two together for me. My own Christian faith found illumination through experiencing CFIDS firsthand after five years of misconceptions had accrued through watching my wife deal with the illness. In the process I found that knowing someone with this hidden disease, however close that person may be, and having it oneself are worlds apart. And because of the first-person perspective that the illness has afforded, my understanding of my faith and my whole sense of spirituality have been permanently reconfigured.

THE ILLNESS PERSPECTIVE

When I was a kid, a time-honored method for responding to an insult was to throw one's accuser's insult back in his face with the comeback, "Takes one to know one!"—usually said with an obvious smirk. Thus, if one was called a "stupid idiot" (disregard the redundancy factor), the "takes one to know one" retort gave one a measure of satisfaction, however temporary it might have been in the course of the conflict.

Underlying that particular rejoinder is a truth tacitly agreed upon by old and young alike. It is the conviction that one cannot really know and understand what a particular circumstance is like without firsthand experience. The same idea is captured in the well-worn admonition, "Before you judge another person, walk a mile in his shoes." It is a way of acknowledging that firsthand experience gives one the required credentials to speak to the needs and concerns of other individuals who share one's circumstances. This principle is central to the approach of Alcoholics Anonymous, as indeed it is for numerous other organizations geared toward helping those with a specific problem or need.

CFIDS is now a firsthand illness for me. It is not some abstraction that involves textbook symptoms and treatments. It is the pain I feel in my muscles and joints, the confusion that clouds my thinking every minute of every day, the weakness and fatigue that have caused me to reluctantly acknowledge thousands of times, "I just can't do that anymore." This knowledge could not have been gained in any other way except to experience the disease wreaking havoc within my own mind and body.

I can unreservedly make such a statement because for the five years that my wife had the illness and I did not, I failed to comprehend her pain and suffering and I sorely misjudged her uncountable times. I simply could not get away from thinking that if she only tried harder or exerted a bit more willpower, then she could break free from the constraints of CFIDS, get up out of bed, and get on with life. That she had an illness was obvious to me, but I also thought that it disabled her because of some weakness of personality and that she could overcome it if she only put her mind to it. I had determined that she simply lacked what used to be called "gumption." In short, I believed that the illness was really her fault (or at least that remaining ill indefinitely could be blamed on her).

Although I made a noble attempt to be empathic, it was more as a matter of principle than anything else. My sympathy was abstract and thus shallow, and I lacked the most basic understanding of what the illness does to affect every system within the body. I had only the vaguest idea of what my wife Louise was going through until I began to experience the unbelievably debilitating symptoms myself.

Getting back to anthropology, the point to consider here is that each and every person relates to the world through his or her own life experiences. Those experiences help to frame a personalized world-view that serves as a kind of template for interpreting the beliefs and behaviors of others. In my case, I had no experience of a chronic illness and took for granted a level of health that is foreign and all but forgotten to people with CFIDS (PWCs). Simply put, I was unable to envision a reality in which strength would not return with rest, in which sleep would not come despite utter exhaustion, in which thinking remained on a permanently impaired level, and in which issues of pain dictated every movement and activity. It was as though Louise was telling me that she lived in a universe where Newtonian physics did not apply, where objects fell upward and not down. My sense of logic recoiled, leaving me questioning not only her experience but her very character.

My love for my wife only clouded the issue. This person whose life was finely interwoven into my own was telling me something that just did not add up with my forty years of experience (nor, I might add, did it add up with my hopes that we might actively share the next forty together). Louise's every hint that she was feeling a bit better was interpreted by me as, "Finally she's getting better!" And her every downturn in health elicited in me a disheartening mixture of frustration and anger. I was frustrated that no significant progress could be measured after years of pain and struggle for us both, and I longed to get back the wife of my youth. The anger, however, was ultimately rooted in the unfounded notion that she could have gotten better if only she really tried. So there I dwelt in my ignorance, doubling Louise's burden whenever I chided her regarding my unmet needs or the perceived needs of our children.

My heart did begin to soften somewhat as the years mounted, giving way to admiration for the way Louise dealt with her unfortunate circumstances. She did not dwell in self-pity nor attempt to convince others of just how much suffering she was enduring. Rather, she matter-of-factly informed people of her condition and left the reacting to them. She saved her energy for the important things: collecting information on the illness to bring the family doctor up to speed on effective treatment of symptoms; finding ways to maintain a positive mental outlook; cooking one meal each day around which our family could maintain some semblance of normality.

Although impressed by her approach to her disability, the real insights only began to emerge after CFIDS "called my number." The illness had slowly but decidedly taken me prisoner, and like a jungle traveler caught in a pit of quicksand, my condition only worsened the more I struggled against it. I had been trapped in the very quagmire that I thought Louise could have willed herself out of. Now, on days when I lie inert upon the couch, crabby and unable to even attend to my own needs, she gives me the compassionate, knowing glance that I, in my prior state of ignorance and inexperience, was never able to offer her.

Many CFIDS sufferers have had the humiliating experience of friends, family, and even physicians telling them, in so many words, that the illness is all in their heads. Lack of sufficient research about the illness has led to a relative paucity of publications and media coverage regarding it. And the name doesn't help. Many people develop an impression of CFIDS from mere hearsay, or even worse, from opportunistic comedians and ill-informed journalists. This situation too often leads to gross misunderstanding about what constitutes the disease and how it affects those disabled by it. And doctors are not immune to the intolerance that such misinformation generates.

There is no way to describe how disheartening it is to hear someone who knows little about CFIDS say: "Oh, everybody gets tired. You just need to get up and get a move on." It is at times such as these that PWCs wish for the proverbial magic wand that would allow their disparagers the opportunity to spend but one day "in their shoes." Still, one can hardly blame nonsufferers for their ignorance. It is simply not possible to know what CFIDS or any other illness is really like unless one experiences it firsthand. Certain kinds of knowledge can only be gained through firsthand suffering; and common suffering, in turn, has the power to bind people together like nothing else can.

DISABILITY'S DOUBLE LENS

Viewing the world through the perspective of a chronic illness gives rise to a paradox. The pain, suffering, and isolation that illnesses such as CFIDS produce can cause sufferers to see the world in an overly negative light. Pain and suffering can easily obscure the good things in life, causing many people to give up the will to live from the grief and despair wrought by chronic pain and disability. Yet, conversely, those who suffer hardship and illness often gain a clearer and more accurate view of life and what is important in it—a spiritual perspective, if you will—than do those who live their days in relative health and happiness.

I readily admit that my disablement via CFIDS has brought to the surface all that is nasty and negative in my personality. It is as though I've undergone a "Jekyll to Hyde" personality change. For me the illness has made it all but impossible to express those qualities that I once considered admirable. Now so many of my interactions with others are characterized by irritability, frustration, and a resignation that I don't have the energy to take a real concern in them. I suppose this comes as no surprise in that there is a direct relationship between the way one feels (happy, sad, sick, tortured) and the way one relates to others.

Serious and unrelenting illness can easily cause one to be downright mean-spirited, no matter how devout a person may be or how affable his or her personality. Everyone has a snapping point. And that point can be reached by simply making one very uncomfortable for an extended period of time.

Elie Wiesel, in his poignant book *Night,* relates an unforgettable example of what can happen when one reaches the breaking point in the human spirit.[1] On an overcrowded Nazi train packed full of desperate and starved Jews being hauled between concentration camps, Wiesel witnessed a young man, hungry and freezing, beat his own father to death in order to get at a crust of bread that had been tossed into the open transport cattle wagon. Wiesel understood the utter desperation that prompted such an act by a young man whose cultural and religious heritage would, under normal circumstances, have led him to show great honor and respect toward his father. Wiesel knew the pain and suffering the young man was experiencing because the writer, along with his own father, was also crammed into that boxcar. The awful incident, and the many to follow, would give Wiesel great insights into human nature and the value of human life—insights that even today he is still called upon to share among world bodies attempting to curb mounting hatred and violence worldwide. Both the horrendous act of the young man and Wiesel's deep reflections came out of their common sufferings. Impulsive violence and fruitful wisdom found rooted in the same soil.

Who could confidently say that he would not do the same as the young prisoner if forced into those desperate and inhumane conditions? I, myself, harbor no illusions that I could have fared any better than the desperate son. I only thank God that he has not put me in such a position, for I shudder to think how I would respond. Take away what makes each person comfortable and secure and the very worst aspects of our human nature easily rise to the surface.

And CFIDS has done that very thing to me and to many who suffer its insidious power to disfigure body, mind, and soul. It has unraveled my spiritual smugness. The unrelenting and very palpable physical and psychological suffering has confined me within a zone of negativity most hours of the day. On occasion it has driven me to hate those I love, to openly curse God and those around me, and to loathe my very life. There has been more than one instance in which suicide seemed the only way to end the unbearable and unrelenting pain and suffering. Yet, fortunately, God does not keep me in that place for long, knowing that I cannot long bear up under its intensity.

It is only through grace that I have not succumbed to those suicidal impulses. During such occasions, the interventions of physicians and medications have proved virtually useless. As the scripture promises, I have not been forced to bear more anguish than I can handle (although the envelope has certainly been pushed and pushed hard). Yet, somehow, through all the pain and turmoil a measure of insight and understanding has emerged. I know myself better now, my faults and strengths. And I can understand the plight of others better as well, my wife foremost among them. The understanding that eluded me prior to CFIDS has now become excruciatingly clear. It is a kind of forced knowledge, gained through the medium of suffering.

PAIN AND FAITH

Bearing pain and suffering with a noble spirit has often been thought of as a bread-and-butter characteristic of devout Christians. It is all but expected of us. And indeed, many people throughout the ages, Christian and otherwise, have borne life's pain and suffering nobly. The numerous martyrs of the Church are evidence that some people are able to sustain their high character even through the most extreme forms of suffering. But their experience is the exception and, I believe, must be the result of a special dispensation of grace that bears them up through their heroic moments.

I do not wish to detract from such examples of faith in the midst of suffering. But the kind of mundane suffering that many disabled PWCs face is in a way more difficult to bear. It is the day-in-and-day-out, unrelenting pain that serious illness and disability inflict. There is no respite and no escape. And the ridicule of an unacknowledged illness only adds salt to the wound. This kind of suffering requires more than a moment's grit and grace. It requires a sustained battle against a ubiquitous but unseen foe. It requires a strength that has nothing to do with physics. The struggle has made me appreciate that even a low level of sustained pain and suffering will grow in an exponential trajectory, so that sooner or later even the most iron will and noble spirit must break, barring God's constant intervention.

My immersion in the pain and disability caused by CFIDS has driven me to reevaluate my whole system of personal beliefs. In this soul searching I've come to realize that a biblically-based understanding of faith must run contrary to the popular notion that spirituality is a means to immunize oneself against hardship and illness. I've discovered that religious faith is not a convenience that can be used to salve unwanted bruises in an otherwise happy-go-lucky life. Rather, biblical faith offers a perspective that applies to every aspect of life, including the inevitable suffering and travail that most people face at some juncture in their life's journey. Such faith engenders an inner knowledge that can help to put suffering in correct perspective. But as is the case with me and CFIDS, faith in God does not necessarily eliminate the source of the suffering. The Apostle Paul and his "thorn in the flesh" experience echoes this difficult truth. What faith does, however, is to change the way one looks at suffering by shedding a purposeful light upon an otherwise cruel and meaningless experience.

I will not for a minute pretend that I have anything but a tenuous grasp on this most difficult topic. It almost goes without saying that any serious consideration of the theological implications of pain and suffering is bound to leave some deep and unresolvable paradoxes. But what is of major concern to me is the many misconceptions surrounding traditional religious views of the interplay between faith and suffering. There is a tendency to place too much emphasis on a person's ability to will himself or herself out of pain and despondency. For this reason I think it vitally important to reemphasize the fact that a person's ability to sustain positive character traits in the midst of suffering has little to do with self-achievement, willpower, or some kind of superior psychological makeup.

Our current understanding of neuroscience clues us in on the fact that brain chemistry plays a key role in how each person perceives and responds to pain. The level of pain tolerance any one person can withstand is to a very large degree a function of that person's distinctive brain chemistry (my two children lie at opposite ends of the spectrum here). What creates mild discomfort for one person can be excruciating pain for another depending upon one's chemical makeup. One often hears this phenomenon referred to today in terms of a person having a high or low "pain threshold." It boils down to recognizing that humans represent a great deal of genetic variability that plays itself out in an awesome display of personality types. We are not Christmas cookies, differentiated only by a few colors and shapes.

Where does that leave boasting? Or for that matter, admonishing or belittling those who succumb to pain sooner than we might? It makes tolerance for pain more a function of biology than of chiseled character. I am not saying that there is no room for a person's will to operate within the givens of biochemistry. But I am saying that the differing limits of tolerance for pain and suffering are primarily determined by one's biochemistry—something for which none of us can take much credit. CFIDS sufferers know this fact because of the way antidepressants and other drugs can for some dramatically lessen pain and disability through a simple altering of brain chemistry. Aspirin works on the same principle.

So much for spirituality—at least the kind associated with being cheery in the midst of suffering. The spiritual person is the one who displays compassion toward those who suffer simply because there is suffering. It has nothing to do with how much of one's own pain can be borne and everything to do with how much of another's hardship one can help to alleviate, especially through the miracle of empathic support. Mother Teresa at work in Calcutta, not the bearded mystic who sleeps upon a bed of nails, exemplifies true spirituality.

Jesus, so far as I know, never called any sufferer he met a "cry-baby" or told anyone to just "suck it up and get on with life." And this despite his own immense capacity ro tolerate pain, evident in his concern for those around him as he said his final farewells upon that diabolic implement of human torture: concern that included seeking forgiveness for the Roman soldiers who drove home those fateful nails. Yet most of us have the simpleminded habit of thinking that everyone around us should be able to bear up as we ourselves can. "If I can do it, why can't you?" is our cultural modus operandi.

It is not unreasonable to expect that empathy and support for the suffering of others has to be based at least in part on an intellectual understanding of what those others are going through. Most people need to be knowledgeable about the effects of an illness before they can offer sympathy. Recognizing this fact means that those of us who suffer from a disability have a responsibility to inform others about our condition if we expect an understanding or sympathetic response. Of course, the facts do not always speak for themselves. In spite of ample evidence to the contrary, some people will simply prefer to believe that CFIDS and other serious disabilities are nothing more than depression and hysteria. In my opinion, such people find that it serves their own purposes better to think that way. They are mere opportunists.

HOPE SPRINGS ETERNAL

For PWCs, as for those disabled by the innumerable other conditions that afflict humankind, there is no single generalized experience of the illness. There are, in fact, as many experiences as there are people. And for me that experience is couched within the context of a faith for which the themes of suffering and firsthand experience are central.

Suffering happens. It is just part of life. And according to Christian theology, it is not always the consequence of bad or "sinful" choices. Sometimes it is just the price of the ticket for being human. This mystery has prompted people of faith down through the ages to reserve judgment against those who suffer, offering instead support and a sense of dignity to those who endure hardship and disability.

This very understanding was what I was unable to offer to my wife and other PWCs until I became one of them. Until I unwillingly moved from the realm of the healthy to the disabled, I could not offer a level of understanding that was even close to adequate. In the process of becoming disabled, I also came to recognize anew how central the Incarnation is to my Christian faith. The disability of CFIDS has illuminated the fact that God's participation in the human endeavor means that his concern for human suffering is real; that is, it is grounded, so to speak, in firsthand experience. After Jesus, compassion could no longer be just a platonic notion, an abstraction built on clayless feet. It had become utterly tangible. Immanuel (God with us) is now for me more than just a Yuletide name for Christ.

I believe that my own life has now come to better reflect this incarnational perspective. Through my own visitation of the world of CFIDS, I have become able to truly understand my wife and her ongoing plight. And I realize that compassion and support, not criticism and skepticism, are the proper responses to offer to her and to all those whose lives have been devastated by disease and disability. Through the long and tortured process I have been learning the importance of not judging those whose lives I don't understand.

Some have theorized that divine compassion could have been expressed through means other than a firsthand experiencing of the human condition. But apparently my understanding of and compassion toward PWCs required it. I needed to feel the pain in order to grasp the gravity of the situation. I would not wish the circumstances of this awful knowledge on anyone else. That would only constitute cruelty. Rather, I sincerely hope that others might find another avenue to knowledge than the one I had to take. Yet at times I do despair that the plight of those broadsided by CFIDS cannot be taken seriously enough without some level of experiencing the illness. Perhaps one has to be in the "cattle car" to really understand. Let's hope that time will prove me wrong.

It is my firm belief that, in spite of a tendency to consider ourselves enlightened, we humans—all of us—are a shortsighted lot. We see through a glass dimly. We often fumble around in the darkness of our own self-concern, causing more harm than good to those in need about us. But I am not a pessimist despite all the misunder-standing that exists about CFIDS and the destructive grip it has on too many lives. Hope and not despair seems somehow at hand. Perhaps this is because my faith and my experience with the illness have underscored the fact that good can come from evil, and that suffering can be redemptive. This hard-won perspective gives me strength of soul for the moment, and hope for a future in which ignorance about CFIDS will eventually be transformed into effective treatment. I know that suffering will not be eliminated in this life, but I do hold fast to the belief that healing and wholeness can be resurrected from its darkened tomb.

NOTE

1. Weisel, Elie. *Night.* New York: Bantam Books, 1986, pp. 95-96. Translated from the French by Stella Rodway.

PART VI:
LOVE AND ALLIANCE

Chapter 25

CFIDS—A Love Poem

Stacey Montgomery

You're a vampire, or at least, I wish that you were
you lead me through graveyards,
where stones like old teeth thrust out of the moldy soil,
and the marble is wrought with the litany of forgotten transgressions
you embrace me in the endless midnight of your bedroom,
and I tilt my head back for you, opening to your hunger,
I want you to drink, to put your mouth to my rhythms and swallow,
I want you to drink me dry, to be healed and restored by my waters,
you don't walk like a sick person, you stride like a runner,
lean and strong, and I want to see you run beneath the moon,
as fast as the wind that you have blown through my empty places
But in the morning you are even more tired,
I am tasty but I do not sustain you,
my blood is a warm and salty river,
but it is not a solution

In the darkness, all sunlight arrested, I trace the meridians of your
    body,
like the ley lines that run past stone circles in ancient grassy fields,
they glow softly against your skin,
flowing with the power that fills you,
I can feel it like heat on my face when you are close,
too much ever to feel sorry for you, or to think you are weak,
but it is a mystery to me where it all goes,
because you are always so weary

You are not the vampire, but there is one here someplace,
drinking your strength, like millions of tiny bats swarming in your
    blood,
sneaking up on helpless platelets and draining them,
leaving them stunned in the back alleys behind your lymph nodes,
where the uniformed leukocytes scratch their heads and say
But, she still has her mitochondria, so robbery wasn't a motive

You pulse with energy, but it's all on your skin and not inside you,
I have seen you run your hands over your body,
your fingers tracing the lines of power that flow across you,
you read to me in bed, your fingers sliding across your shape,
like all your secrets are written on your skin,
and you read them back to me in Braille,
when I press myself against you I wonder if the arcs and lines will
    transfer onto me,
so that I am marked by lambent cursive like yours, but backwards,
and we would be joined in the same alphabet
but even then my strength would not flow through those paths into
    you,
you are not a vampire, and I am not a healing well, or cut from a
    unicorn's brow,
nor recombined with a eureka,
I have so little to offer you
when we sit together in the sad sterility and flat light of emergency
    waiting rooms,
you and me and the mystery that has stolen so much from you

I wrap you up in my skin
paler than yours because I am like you, undead and unalive,
like a character who dies before the beginning of the story
and only appears as other people's memories,
I am the empty space in a universe that is everything else but me,
you can be safe here and find words in that void,
words you have forgotten or misplaced,
names for things you didn't realize you needed so badly,
I wonder if you'll find a thesaurus glistening on my skin
and write it all down in your notebooks for later or just read me aloud,
your face dead in the harsh blue light of an all night diner,

or blanched by theater spotlights as your purpled lips pronounce and
    shape me,
You and I are always on stage,
writing dialogue for each other, and prompting lines and directions,
without your directions I would be lost
for you are like a labyrinth that I must walk, hoping always to find the
    center,
like a story that is never quite finished,
like a long night in the broken smile of a churchyard with my throat
    exposed,
waiting for the vampire and her magic kiss,
like just making a space for us, and the darkness, and the mystery.

Chapter 26

What's a Mother to Do?

Gloria Kartiganer

My daughter Lily, who runs off to Central America to help after a devastating hurricane; who writes a paper on humanitarian aid to read at a significant international relations conference; who picks up dead animals to respectfully place them on the side of roads and cover them with leaves; who investigates how the local hospital is dealing with non-English-speaking immigrants and reports what is lacking to the city authorities; who stops to offer help to a woman on the street who is being threatened by a loudly enraged man; who makes special visits to chat with those homeless who sit begging in the doorways with their children; who stands up in the movie theater as soon as the film is over and boldly asks the audience to tell the management that the advertising poster for the film in the display window is sexist; who cares both empathically and thoughtfully for the ill, the emotionally hurt, the jailed (this is the short list)—this dynamo daughter is now physically downed with a mysterious and highly disabling illness called chronic fatigue immune dysfunction syndrome (CFIDS).

Mostly I listen. Last week was one of the hardest weeks. Long-distance on the phone, she shamefully tells me she is so deeply exhausted she could not even brush her teeth for three days. Something drops into my stomach and spits rays of burning fire there. I listen further. She has been able to take a walk only once in the last two weeks. I try to numb out so I won't cry as the suicide wonderings softly spill from her. I hear how emotionally fragile she is from the bizarre symptoms of this illness. I breathe and remember she does not always feel this way. In order to go on, with another part of my brain I reach for hope, for an image of her well again. After such calls I cry to release the hurt so I can return to wholeness. By necessity I've learned a way of meditating that fills me with energy to recover from the painful talks, and there's the gym, or yoga, and the walks up the hill, and those who listen to me cry, and a caregivers support group I irregularly attend. I am lucky to be able to bounce back from grief in an hour, or a day, or two days. It used to take longer. Sometimes, if I sit quietly, I can recover in a few minutes.

I listen for her sake, because I want her to be able to share this journey that isolates her. And for my sake. My urge to know her is so strong. She is a role model for me as I share her victories. Losing one career, she has found a new one, painting watercolors. She's talented in it. Several pieces were sold this year. Her persistence is productive and rather astonishing. Her romances are unique and surprising too, since she has such limited ability to come into contact with the public.

A challenge for me is to overcome my selling of New Age advice, as she calls it. I have lots of advice to give, which she does not want. She fiercely insists that I not tell her yet again to stretch or do mild yoga on days she cannot take a walk. I have put a sign on my phone, *No More Advice*, but I don't read it. The illness has been going on too long. What part of this battle is mine? To learn patience, to respect her choices? Can I master my end of it? And what more can I do?

Early on, there were trips to doctors. (Why don't the lungs heal from pneumonia? Why don't the antibiotics work? Why do the wrists act like they have carpal tunnel syndrome, when she hadn't done repetitive work?) And going to talks together or separately, desperate for useful information. (What about getting to sleep? What causes the disease?) And the minimal physical support of driving, cleaning, shopping. Now, in the fifth year, I am no longer in the same part of the country. In the awful days, there is almost daily telephone listening. I mostly enjoy this part, I so much like who she is; she's almost always interesting. Then, I get crushed listening to the cries. This happens when there are extended periods, weeks or worse yet months, of bad spells; and the suicide talks, to which I'm almost getting accustomed.

Then, last year, the fifth year of illness, I gave her my house to live in, a serious loss of income for me at a critical financial period. She had been wandering around for years, living in one cheap place after another, negotiating with landlords about her needs relative to paint fumes, sawdust, money, and accessible house entrances. With my recent move to another state, and new career building, I have erratic work and a limited income. However, I am so much calmer and breathe easy knowing she is in a safe and beautiful house. Not only can't she get kicked out again or move, but she can have the quiet she needs regularly. It is exhausting for her to be with others. She needs often to retreat behind a veil and be in the solitude the illness demands of her.

I thought this charming old Vermont hayloft house of mine, with garden and trees, would allow her to get well. But *no*, this year has been one of the worst for her physically. How can that be? It is not supposed to be like that. Why has the stability of the house not worked to aid her body to heal? Should she have had the house years ago, at the beginning? Would that have helped? Again, I take comfort knowing, though her physical health has not improved, she loves to be in this charming old house, with the wood ceilings, which she has lushly decorated with plants and candlesticks.

Caretaking, with my daughter and others in the family too, has taken a front seat in how I've used my time recently. It has been changing my point of view about how I value myself. I have been very attached to judging myself by my work accomplishments. I have been gradually leaving that arena. I am putting first affairs of my heart. My intention is to approach every act or moment in an open, full-hearted way. Daily, I succeed and fail at this. Even when I am hurting from my pain or hers, I try to center my energy in my heart and radiate the energy out, warmly, kindly, to myself and others. I am valuing myself now as a good sister, mother, friend, rather than by my "job." My accomplishments are direct, person to person, rather than through the role of teacher, theater director, and so on. Truthfully, I'd like to give up judging altogether. Maybe soon.

In my daydreams I see Lily able to socialize, dance, think clearly, sleep peacefully, doing the work she loved before the Unknown snatched her energy and left her lying limp as a Dali clock. In her worse times I have consulted a psychic and an astrologer for comfort. She will get well, maybe by the end of 2000 or soon after! I want to believe. I will test their other predictions in the upcoming months. Am I desperate?

I am exhausted. Differently than she is. Am I exhausted from the ache of watching her, who is tied to my heart, dredge up the courage it takes to overcome the limitations and face the day, every single day?

Am I depressed from hopelessness as I watch the sixth year in which she has periods in which she pushes herself to put one foot in front of the other because going for a walk is a heroic act? I look around and find no one who will award her with a purple heart for the month of fake energy she produced to find the cheapest responsible car she could find. It is discouraging as I imagine her effort merely to *think* because her thought is stopped by the walls of a recurrent brain fog. With clouded brain, how can she figure out what to do?

I get discouraged. My heart cracks again and then expands again as I see her overcome the many humiliations of *needing* from others. Will she learn to surrender to needing without feeling humiliation? What kind of values does our culture promote when needing has to be so humiliating? I am tired from merely witnessing, and I don't have the illness. Is this the role for me? To listen and witness? With compassion? And then to be the outside voice calling to her, "Hold on! Remember, this too will pass"?

Of course there is the desire to sell my New Age advice. I have lots of advice to give. Which she does not want. It slips through my mouth into her ear anyway. So she reminds me. When she asks, I am to give advice. There is still good humor in this dance of ours, but sometimes she gets frustrated with me.

What is confusing for me are the times when I am sad or grieving or depressed. I can't tell—is it because of her or me? I also have a life full of its own ups and downs, including stresses such as other major family illnesses, lack of productive work, financial challenges. I have learned I sometimes get confused about what's what. I don't look carefully enough at myself and how I give in to despair and disappointment. Recently, with several people in my circle of family and friends very ill, and my work life at a standstill, I just caved in, drained. This month I am rebuilding myself with rest and peacefulness and more play.

I ask you, who also love the ones pushed out of simple daily ordinary society (an often banal society, which suddenly seems extremely precious when you can't have it), what is a mother to do? I witness her. With her small parcel of energy she produces for herself in many arenas, extraordinarily misunderstood and even blamed by government agencies and friends alike. Unable to get much relief for symptoms that to me appear to be a jumble of multiple sclerosis, flu, brain malfunction, low blood pressure, body exhaustion, and the additional exhaustion that poverty creates when one is forced to argue with oneself and others about pennies for necessities. I *witness,* is that what you do? Also, I have given her my money and a good place to live.

Because my antennae are out, I have met many new, interesting people with CFIDS and its relatives, fibromyalgia and environmental illness. I have loved some of them too; in a few cases just from poignant meetings on the phone. Most special is Jane, my confidante, to whom I trust my inner world. She has wisdom of the mind and heart. For two weeks she gave me a place to live. I heard her nights, with fitful sounds of rage and cries from the muscle pain of fibromyalgia. As one of my new close friends, she is a gift to me. Then there is Helena. I traveled a thousand miles to help Helena, frail in body, but iron of spirit, so she could relocate from cold Minnesota to the warm Southwest. Among the primitive red cliffs, I spent June cooking and driving her for experimental ozone treatments. Who knew if they would work? However, we discovered worms in her stools. Live worms. I drove them in a vial to a parasitologist in another state and left them on her porch as I was directed to do. I want artistic Helena and gifted Jane and gentle Daniel from Korea, and Peter, who is losing his sight, and politically savvy Robert—I want them well. Not just my daughter; I want all those suffering to be well.

How to make that happen? The helplessness of it all drains me. I don't know what to do. I am searching for direction. Do what? And I notice I am also searching for the energy to act. I want to be part of a march (not a creep) toward making the illness respectable in the eyes of society, and more important, finding a cure. I have been looking for where I fit in what seems like a huge CFIDS abyss. This essay is a call! I am looking for the able-bodied ones who love those who are ill so I can join you. I want to find you and tell you and ask you, can we dream together? Can we move this stone together and get strength from one another? Those ill with these diseases do not have the energy to do this, and neither do I alone. What I know for sure is I can't do it alone. I have tried. It's much too hard on me to get doors shut in my face regularly. I need the joyful energy of an enthusiastic community. Together it could be meaningful and even fun in the sharing.

So, please, let's talk.

Chapter 27

Dating CFIDS

Andrew Corriveau

I have always been a film buff and, in fact, always imagined my life as a film, with a pensive background score and a beautiful, witty costar appearing sometime around my middle age. So, when I met her on that too-green afternoon, at a backyard party of some mutual friends, I thought she was perfect—funny and bright and attractive and creative.

I didn't know that she had taken various medications, two packets of multiple B vitamins, coenzyme Q-10, and numerous other supplements just to haul herself to this rare social occasion. I didn't know she hadn't been to a party in three years. I didn't know that every time she left her house, she had to be an actress of the highest caliber. I simply thought her laugh was enchanting. I liked the way she took more dip than chips, and when she picked around her food plate, managed to eat all of the dip and only some of the chips. Such caloric indulgence in public seemed to indicate bravado. I liked her hair, which was long and partially tucked under an artistic hat. When I asked her what she did for a living she was vague, mumbled something about being a musician, and said she worked in disability rights. Great, I thought to myself with admiration—an artist and social activist. She was pretty, too, with dark, sunken eyes.

When she seemed to be leaving, I thrust my business card into her hand and told her I would love to talk more. She glanced down at the card—as if she had already forgotten my name—and said, "I enjoyed meeting you too, Andrew."

I was pleased and surprised to hear from her the very next night. She explained she had left the party early because she wasn't feeling well, so I mentioned that a twenty-four-hour flu was going around my office. Then, after some reluctance, she admitted she had been severely ill for five years. She had chronic fatigue syndrome.

"Oh," I answered, taken aback. "You mean what Keith Jarrett has?"

I was a collector of jazz and blues, and I had recently read about the legendary jazz musician's struggle with the illness, how he was so sick he couldn't even *listen* to music for a whole year. My thoughts digressed and I imagined taking her to my favorite local club on a good night, maybe when A'Lelia Rain was singing blues. My date would look, in a streamlined black dress, like Holly Hunter in the movie *Living Out Loud,* hip and sexy, and she would teach me about love and heroic independence and I would nod compassionately. A'Lelia would sing about salvation, and I would feel like a kind of salvation, how I rescued her from her home and swept her right into the ancient healing waters of the blues. But this was merely a fantasy—it never happened.

Rule Number 1: There is no salvation, only salvaging. When you date someone with CFIDS, you will imagine yourself as her salvation, if even for a second. You will briefly think yourself to be courageous and open-minded and maybe a little heroic. Remember, this is your ego talking. You will think, "She doesn't look that sick so she must be over the worst part of it." You will fully believe her recovery is imminent. In other words, your attraction may be contingent on change, a change she has been hoping for and praying for and wanting for five years. At first, you probably won't consider what she has to teach you. You won't realize what you can learn from her about the fragility of health and the tenuousness of every moment. You won't realize that she can teach you to be an alert scavenger of life, abandoning your fantasy of being rescued from your mundane existence and instead learning to salvage the beauty in pedestrian reality.

"Actually," she answered when I asked her when we could meet again, "I can only get out unpredictably [which was a huge understatement—she was bedridden a great deal of the time]. Do you want to come over here for tea? And please don't wear anything scented. I have chemical sensitivities."

Rule Number 2: You will shower with baking soda, per her instructions, because all of your shampoos and soaps have chemical fragrances. You will begin to feel inconvenienced, like that time you dated the single mother with an eight-year-old daughter. The daughter scowled when you walked into the room. You thought the mother coddled the daughter. You thought the daughter needed tough love. You were jealous whenever the daughter ended your dates too early, even though you offered to drive the baby-sitter home. As the baby-sitter chattered away about her new true love—a guy who played bass in a band—you wanted to tell her that real love involves irritating compromises. You wanted to tell her that the bass is the instrument of four-fingered Neanderthals and she shouldn't be so happy after making a measly twenty-five dollars for spending the evening with a scowling child. You will think of the illness as another scowling daughter who has nothing to do with you.

"It's no big deal for me," I said about her illness, which is of course like saying a woman's child is no big deal, which of course indicates that I have never changed a diaper. My fantasy started to unwind.

Rule Number 3: You will feel duped by the collision of fantasy and reality. You will show up at her house, and she will pretend not to be exhausted by the effort of making the tea and laying out the store-bought cookies. You will have a great, engaging conversation, but she will look a little gaunt. The conversation will be so good that you will forget she is sick, but *she* won't forget. Later, you will learn that she never forgets, that the hideous adulterer inside her never lets her fully be with you. She never has a minute without flulike symptoms, pain, and unbelievable exhaustion. In your period of forgetfulness, though, you will fantasize about stroking her hair, reading the Sunday paper together, going out to concerts, and making her laugh just to see the creases around her mouth. Then she will say, "I have to kick you out. If I don't rest I'm going to collapse." Her statement will hit you like lightning, but then you will notice how pale she is, the strain in her voice. Why can't she be healthy? She is almost, practically, what you've been looking for . . .

The first time I touched her I thought I would break. She was so strong in her apparent fragility, though her muscle tone was almost gone. Her skin was pale and smooth. I wanted to be the courageous one. I wanted to be William Hurt in *Children of a Lesser God,* making love to a disabled woman in a fuzzy, Hollywood way that made *him* look heroic. I wanted to be able. Instead, I felt a vague sense of endangerment. I felt afraid of tiny, invisible, paranoid things—minute pathogens. I felt thrown back to pubescent ignorance, when bodies are surging with change and hormones and unpredictability and the boy is supposed to be in charge. Her flesh was the war-torn country where I was about to come of age. Or destroy others. Or die. I was terrified of this thing inside of her, this landmine of an illness that nobody could detect and nobody could understand. Then, I shamefully balked. I said it was late and I should go home. On the walk to my apartment, every noise jolted me, but my body felt virile and alive in the night air. I wondered if she was too sick to take walks. I wanted something small and simple, to walk in the cold air and hold her hand.

I later found out that she was too sick to walk around the block on most days. For everything she did, the illness harshly punished her.

Rule Number 4: You will feel afraid. You will feel afraid that she is contagious. You will feel afraid that she might burden you. You will feel afraid that you won't be as strong as she seems to be. You will be afraid that she won't keep up with you. You will be afraid of being the weaker sex, since she is too sick to take care of you. You will feel afraid of hurting her. You will feel afraid of being a jerk to her. After all, she can't help her situation. You will feel guilty. You will wish you could give some money to charity and forget the whole thing. But then you will remember what you see in her—courage, honesty, warmth, humor, insight, compassion.

The first time we slept together I realized I had a lot to learn about sex. "Sex is not acquisition but barter," she said. "Everything is a negotiation." She told me what would leave her in bed for weeks. She told me what she liked. She asked me what made my body feel good. She knew about comfort and danger, how they can abut each other in the nether regions of the body. She knew how to find them, coax them out, talk to them. Then she had to stop suddenly and asked me if I could get her a drink of water. She managed to prop herself up on a pillow. It was only then that I realized she was too sick to get up. "Sorry," she said, and seemed a bit ashamed.

I later learned that sex, which she loved and which exhilarated both of us at the time, made her feel like she was dying. I hated this. I hated having to negotiate everything with her illness, that tyrant. It felt so unfair.

Rule Number 5: You will realize that your fantasy of life has always involved fairness. You have fantasized for years about what you deserve—the perfect home, the perfect state of fitness, a perfect partner. You have felt entitled to all of these things. You have preferred the notion of them, largely, to reality. No, in fact, you have believed them to be real. You have believed fairness to be real. You will realize there is a fine line between fantasies that preserve and fantasies that detract from experience.

"I really envy your life," she said as I was talking about her illness and she was lying under the covers with me after watching a really bad foreign film where the main characters were bicycling across country with wild abandon.

She admitted, breaking down into tears, that she used to cycle regularly with an old boyfriend. The tires of her bike were cardboard-narrow, racing tires, and she used to burn down Southern country roads leaning down over her handlebars looking over at her boyfriend, who was a misogynistic dolt but beautifully aerodynamic. She was obsessed with her own quadriceps, how strong and toned they were. He didn't leave her because of her illness but her next boyfriend did. She watched her friends go off to law school, to other countries, to adventures. She gave up her job and many of her dreams. She also used to ride horses, work out, keep a garden, carry heavy boxes. All of these abilities vanished overnight.

"I had it all when I got sick," she said. "After years of working to get there, I had just what I wanted. My life was finally right."

But then something in me turned. I wanted attention. My own life wasn't so great. I hated my current job as a journalist for a mediocre paper and didn't feel that good about where my life was going. I felt ungrateful for my own state of angst. I wanted to complain. I wanted to escape. I resented her.

Then I felt frustrated. We had a petty argument and I left.

Rule Number 6: You will deal with difficult struggles that will seem to be about other things, but will be about the illness. You will feel angry at fate and wonder if the relationship is worth it. You haven't been dating that long. You could walk away. It will be hard to separate what is emotional from what is perhaps viral. You will think she is worth the extra work. After all, everyone has drawbacks, and you are not perfect. Or maybe you will think she is not worth it. You will be angry at all the spontaneous adventures you cannot have with her. You want to fly off to Paris, backpack the Appalachian trail, drive all night and into the next day. Perhaps you will break up. Perhaps you will stay. Sometimes, it will feel remarkably similar to other relationships you've had in the past, with the familiar struggles and drama.

Then, maybe, because she is too sick to go out, you will buy some premium ice cream and read to her in bed. You will love the wonderful insularity of your nights together, the intimate banter, how they remind you of childhood thunderstorm afternoons. You will curl up into your mutual microcosm and feel safe and beautiful and warm next to her. You will almost forget she is sick. But she won't forget.

You will think about Billie Holiday's admonition that the blessed child is the one who's "got his own." And you'll visualize yourself at a table alone in your favorite club, looking at other women, but not desiring what you don't already have. And you may realize that you are grateful for what you already have. "Tomorrow," you will think to yourself. "Even if I have to go out alone. I'm going to listen to the blues."

Chapter 28

Sick Sex Revisited

Susan Dion

"Take several platitudes, mix them up with sex and smiles, and call me in six years." Well, six years have passed since I wrote a short, hopeful essay titled "Sick Sex," and I'm checking back. "Sick Sex" pointed out ways to "maintain a desired sexual relationship . . . despite awful illness that cruelly robs in significant areas of life."[1] Since writing it in late 1993, many mouthfuls of simple advice have been swallowed, moderate but frequent doses of humor have been imbibed, and attenuated efforts to keep a sexual life from expiring have continued. I wrote then: "Sex may be of added benefit to people with long-term sickness because it can temporarily (albeit briefly) anesthetize the pain and discomfort of illness." So, what can I add now? Life goes on, in spite of debilitating illness? When you're handed lemons, make lemonade? Hang in there?

When life-changing illness strikes, sometimes the most clichéd, self-evident bits of wisdom act as a lifeline through desperate moments. Hanging on to one's sexuality adds an element of joy in a bleak daily existence. Sex, humor, and platitudes, like illness itself, hide layers of meaning beyond their first-glance obviousness. Platitudes are ubiquitous and easily ridiculed, yet they can be affirming and sustaining. Indeed, their very simplicity often paradoxically masks complex human truths. Sex is common enough, yet it is an enigmatic and spiritual force of life itself. Keeping sexual desire alive and active was important to me, despite a heavy physical cost. Only with hindsight does the audacity of claiming sexuality in the midst of miserable symptoms seem impossibly unrealistic and overly romantic.

"Sick Sex" was full of practical advice on how to manage limitations and decrease the physical toll extracted from lovemaking. I suggested reducing the strenuous elements and adjusting schedules. Avoidance was recommended when other extra efforts were demanded (a doctor appointment or tending to a sick child). Changing attitudes and lowering expectations were perhaps the most emotionally challenging requirements for partners: "Both partners need to gradually accept that less frequent sex will be the norm with sickness. . . . However, learning to cherish one's sexual intimacies within the context of so many constraints can actually improve sexual joy for both healthy and ill persons. It becomes that much more of a treasure." Lastly, paying attention to all forms of tenderness, whispering, holding hands, "gentle hugging, sweet kissing, or passionate touching"—was a key ingredient to ongoing intimacy.

One of my favorite truisms from the early CFIDS years was a variation on the glass that's half empty or half full. As a result of CFIDS, fibromyalgia, cardiac troubles, and other health problems, my glass was 90 percent empty and perhaps 10 percent full. Focusing on the life lost was detrimental to my emotional well-being, so it made sense to somehow appreciate the remains. But how can one be content with 10 percent? This was an arduous struggle for me—to move beyond paralyzing grief and sadness. Somehow I needed to be an agent of change—to reconstruct a meaningful life when it was achingly tough to even brush my teeth or take a bath.

When I wrote "Sick Sex," I'd been severely ill for almost five years. My daily existence was awful. Oppressive flulike symptoms hammered me day and night. It was painful to move, to sleep, to attempt small tasks. My work life was destroyed, my ability to parent was seriously compromised, and my meager stabs at contributing to family life were done while feeling terribly sick. Intellectual labor—writing a sentence or reading a paragraph—was a challenge as words did not make sense, characters and ideas were swiftly forgotten, and a mushy brain received distorted information from the page and pen. Maintaining a sexual relationship was exceedingly difficult, as my libido was poor and intense pain and "flu" were ever-present. But I was (and I remain) fiercely committed to doing my best to be an adequate mom to my two children, Brett and Raena, and a decent companion to Tom, my husband.

Platitudes—as stupid-sounding and simpleminded as many are—somehow got me through each day with their elementary but sound wisdom. Sex helped me feel alive. Now I reread my own advice: "By incorporating sick sex and making it work, a person greedily holds on to one of life's gifts. It is an affirmation of life, rather than another sickness robbery." I still believe, as I wrote then, that "sex offers a deep and mysterious (sacred) joining of two people," that sex "can provide escape, release, pleasure, and profound joy." I once joked to my husband, "Sex or dinner tonight?" as it was evident that only one would be the major goal of the day. His answer didn't surprise me. But what is sick sex exactly? And has my understanding changed since that essay of six years ago?

Honestly describing the barriers to and the costs of keeping sex alive while living with illness is similar to trying to tell a healthy person what it's like to be inside my debilitated body. There is a black hole of inadequate language to capture the actual *feel*. It's somewhat wacky to merge sensual tenderness with nasty symptoms. Contradictions loom large. Too often, the surface of my skin reacts in pain even to a gentle touch. I awake the day after sex with increased stiffness and excessive fibromyalgia pain throughout my body. The overall flulike sickness (fever, night sweats, weakness, foggy brain, etc.) is intensified. Added rest is demanded, as it is in any bad case of the flu. These heavier symptoms may continue for several days. Thus my low-level functioning suffers even more. With determination and careful pacing—before and after—I'm able to get by, but to an outsider sex may seem like a prohibitively expensive extravagance. For me, however, sick sex remains a desired activity; the benefits far outweigh the costs. I refuse to let it go.

Perhaps my most clever insight is a simple one: sick sex is not just about sex. It's about family, love, meaning, purpose, growth, tiny efforts, and more. It's about making choices in illness and in life. It is about coping with the unexpected and adjusting to the unwanted circumstances. It's about dealing with what develops—meeting it head-on—picking oneself up—carrying on despite harsh limitations. And, yes, eventually and ultimately, it is about being an activist survivor and not a passive victim. CFIDS has the capacity to steal everything from us, but only if we give it permission to do so. Yes, illness is destructive but within its aggressive confines, we must choose our paths wisely.

As a couple, my husband and I have faced several significant transitions; we've entered into a new stage with the "empty nest." The obligations of hands-on daily parenting no longer require intensive time and effort, and thus there is more freedom and privacy for us as a twosome. Sadly, we've lost three of our parents. My still-active sixty-eight-year-old father passed away in 1994 after many years of heart disease and several heart attacks. Our mothers died within four months of each other in 1995; my mom's death was especially hard as a swift and furious cancer attacked unexpectedly when she was young and full of teenage spirit and energy. In addition, we've aged and matured as individuals. In other words, life goes on regardless of disabling sickness. If we don't make a commitment to keep (no matter how tentative a grasp) some special parts of life intact, it is our loss. The precious parts rescued and preserved may vary from person to person (painting, friendships, parenting, reading, etc.), but the lessons are the same. It would have been forgivable and understandable for me to forget or neglect sex once illness hit. Weeks would have turned into months and months into years. I'd have a very different story to share, if so.

Looking back over ten and one-half years with disabling CFIDS and other difficult conditions—all following a rotten flu in March 1989—I'm in awe. When I fell ill so suddenly, my son was a high-school junior and my daughter was a fourth grader. At that time, I was a mere thirty-five. I was a young mom who enjoyed her work life and whose income was essential to the family (I taught history and women's studies for a dozen years and directed a women's program for six of those years). I'd earned my bachelor's and master's degrees while balancing my role as parent and provider. And I was approximately 90 percent finished with the writing of my doctoral dissertation. Tom and I had been together for less than four years. We were looking forward to our future. Never in a million thoughts had I ever realistically contemplated living with a vicious sickness that would keep me out of the workforce for years and leave me dependent upon my Social Security Disability for income. Never, no way. How can one comprehend such a reality when strong, energetic, and healthy? Never did I believe in years one, two, three, four, and five that the flu from hell could continue for yet another year. If I had been given this "sentence" in year one or two, I might not have survived. My hold was often too tenuous.

From the vantage point of age forty-six, I am not smug. I recognize what a delicate, fragile web one weaves as she or he reconstructs life with a debilitating illness. Nothing—absolutely nothing— is easy. Slicing a carrot, reading a child's essay, or writing one clear sentence can require extraordinary fortitude and extract a heavy toll with symptoms. So I sit and watch the sorghum grow in the adjacent farm field as I craft a few words in the early weeks of autumn 1999. I'm thankful that my husband and I are still together after more than fourteen years and that I remain close to my daughter and son. I'm now reaping the satisfactions of seeing my children—two kind, balanced, joyful, interesting, diligent young people—come into their own (Raena is a college junior; Brett earned his bachelor's degree and lives and works in New York City). I continue to plod along attempting things bit by bit. And, with great help and endurance, I did complete that dissertation by tackling the remaining small pieces in very short sessions. My defense in late 1991 was modified to take place over two days, rather than the normal one lengthy session. I don't recommend this type of effort to anyone, but I needed the sense of completion. The photos from the university show a thin pale woman looking horribly ill. (I had almost forgotten that I lost about 50 percent of my hair in those initial years of fever and perpetual flu; it came off in clumps in the shower.)

I'm happy to report that I still sleep with my husband. Yes, we share the same bed. Yes, we still find passion and tenderness, despite the chronic pain and symptoms. We're better friends than we were in the 1980s—older, more patient, more accepting of difference. We've benefited from many of the pointers contained in "Sick Sex," but as I reflect I see that one approach appears crucial: "Caring for each other in many small ways throughout the normal pressures of everyday life and the extraordinary circumstances of chronic sickness translates to a better relationship. And it's the everyday love that sustains a commitment to sexual intimacy." "Sick Sex" continues to be requested and reprinted. Perhaps its basic upbeat words provide some comfort and instruction. Perhaps it reiterates the concept that while everything changes, one can hold on to important elements in life. Certainly one's sexual activity undergoes reconstruction—but it can survive and even flourish—similar to other parts of life. So different, so diminished—yet paradoxically full.

NOTE

1. Dion, Susan. "Sick Sex." *Network,* Spring 1994, Connecticut CFIDS Association.

Chapter 29

Long Illness

Ellen Samuels

In the fleshed light
of evening, my face grows thin
beneath your touch.

On our bedside table, grape
hyacinth, black-eyed susan, cut
from the garden; emptied

glass tipped on its side;
paperbacks' furrowed spines.
Each night you kneel

at the tub, squeeze
the cloth over my neck,
aching with heat. I wake

with your hand, in sleep
trembling over
the sill of my back:

unreconciled, holding me here.

"Long Illness" by Ellen Samuels originally appeared in *Contemporary Verse 2,* Summer 1998. Reprinted with permission.

Index